"Finally! The scientific literature on acceptance and commitr. group intervention methods, but through nearly three decades of such studies, no book has been available to walk clinicians through the myriad choice points, barriers, and opportunities presented by ACT in groups. No more. This wonderful and readable volume walks through every relevant area and issue in a way that is wise, evidence-based, and clear. How can you organize an open membership ACT group? What if a group member just wants to tell stories? In area after area and issue after issue, Westrup and Wright have skillfully done the heavy lifting for you. If you're doing ACT in groups, you now have a much easier job: buy the book, read it, and use it."

—**Steven C. Hayes, PhD**, Foundation Professor of Psychology at the University of Nevada, and cofounder of ACT

"This long-awaited book finally provides therapists with the guidance they needed to do ACT in groups. Darrah Westrup and Joann Wright have turned their scientific expertise and clinical wisdom into a wonderfully written text that covers all the key aspects of the psychological flexibility model while addressing the typical pitfalls and advantages of doing ACT in this context. This is an essential read for all therapists doing ACT in groups!"

—**Matthieu Villatte, PhD**, coauthor of *Mastering the Clinical Conversation*

"Life's too short to beat around the bush, so I'm going to be blunt: if you do ACT with groups, or if you wish to start doing so, you need this book. Chockablock full of wisdom and experience from experts in the field, it's not just an optional extra; it's an absolute essential. If you want to help groups of people to discover ACT, and leave them glowing with a sense of vitality and fulfilment, then be smart about it: allow Westrup and Wright to light the way for you."

—**Russ Harris**, author of *The Happiness Trap* and *ACT Made Simple*

"Westrup and Wright have masterfully woven the ACT approach into the group therapy milieu. Contextual behavioral science, the foundation of ACT, suggests the human condition evolved through the blending of two levels of selection: the group and the individual. The ACT community has long endeavored to address the human condition in a way that reduces suffering and improves quality of living by using applied behavioral science to help at the individual level. Thankfully Westrup and Wright are contributing to the applied literature with an eye on utilizing group therapy to direct the therapeutic process in important, valuable directions. *Learning ACT for Group Treatment* highlights advanced ACT topics in a manner accessible for a novice. This pioneering book offers practical exercises for immediate application, and gives incisive examples of how to use them in an ACT-consistent manner. Most importantly, Westrup and Wright created a flexible framework to create unique, impactful group therapy interactions. Highly recommended, even if you are not a group therapist."

—**D.J. Moran, PhD, BCBA-D**, founder of Pickslyde Consulting and the MidAmerican Psychological Institute

"It's here! And it's just what's needed for the therapist looking to do ACT in a group format. For those who have been waiting and asking for a thoughtful and effective guide—including material ranging from brief basics on ACT to utilizing core processes in a powerful and dynamic way in group therapy to supplementary content designed to support its implementation—this is the book for you. Darrah Westrup and Joann Wright have written this manual in a user-friendly fashion. The book is comprehensive in nature, while also maintaining a compassionate clinical voice—felt in both the example dialogue and the overall approach. ACT delivered in the context of group therapy is not only robust, but also helps clients to connect with others in the very human experience of suffering. Westrup and Wright bring these qualities to life. A must-read for those doing or wanting to do ACT in groups."

—**Robyn D. Walser, PhD**, coauthor of *Learning ACT*, *The Mindful Couple*, and *Acceptance and Commitment Therapy for the Treatment of Post-Traumatic Stress Disorder and Trauma-Related Problems*; director of TLConsultation Services; assistant professor at the University of California, Berkeley; and cofounder of the Bay Area Trauma Recovery Clinic

"Brought to us by two ACT master clinicians, *Learning ACT for Group Treatment* is an essential addition to the library of any therapist who uses mindfulness, acceptance, and compassion processes in groups. This book brings the psychological flexibility model to life in the context of group therapy. I am confident that this text can enhance the effectiveness of any of our group-based work. Masterful!"

—**Dennis Tirch, PhD**, coauthor of *The ACT Practitioner's Guide to the Science of Compassion*, and founder of The Center for Compassion Focused Therapy

LEARNING ACT *for* GROUP TREATMENT

AN ACCEPTANCE *and* COMMITMENT THERAPY
SKILLS TRAINING MANUAL *for* THERAPISTS

DARRAH WESTRUP, PhD
M. JOANN WRIGHT, PhD

CONTEXT PRESS
An Imprint of New Harbinger Publications, Inc.

Publisher's Note

This publication is designed to provide accurate and authoritative information in regard to the subject matter covered. It is sold with the understanding that the publisher is not engaged in rendering psychological, financial, legal, or other professional services. If expert assistance or counseling is needed, the services of a competent professional should be sought.

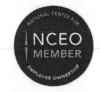
Library of Congress Cataloging-in-Publication Data on file

Printed in the United States of America

24   23   22

10   9   8   7   6   5

Contents

Introduction

We have observed that regardless of theoretical orientation, purpose, means, or setting, facilitators of group therapy—including us—share a firm belief in the therapeutic power of group intervention. If you have had the opportunity to lead or participate in a therapy group, we are willing to bet that you have also witnessed its transformative power. (You also may have experienced the potential challenges of group work—more on that later.) Something powerful occurs in groups. In this book we seek to put forth acceptance and commitment therapy as a treatment that harnesses and optimizes that power.

It seems logical that if we could articulate the change mechanisms at work in group therapy, our clinical skills would be enhanced. If we know what it is that we are doing that works, and why it works, it stands to reason that this would then effectively guide us in session. It could also help prevent us from making moves that might work against what we ultimately are hoping to accomplish.

Over thirty years of applied research suggests that there are certain behavioral processes at work in a therapy group that *can* be articulated. These processes cross over therapist, participant, and setting differences because they pertain to fundamental principles of human behavior. Better yet, these processes can be, and have been, extensively studied, offering substantive support to these mechanisms as vehicles for change.

This book is about a therapy—acceptance and commitment therapy, or ACT—that arose from the research in basic behavioral processes at the heart of both psychological suffering and the ability to flourish despite life's challenges. It is a ground-up therapy developed to target ways in which humans get stuck and to optimize mechanisms of change. While not the only way, it is a highly effective way to help clients move forward in their lives.

We will introduce and work through the therapy as applied in groups with the intention that readers will gain a solid understanding of how to implement ACT in the group setting. We are believers, having found ACT to lend itself particularly well to group therapy. In fact, as Darrah says, ACT in a group setting is like "ACT on steroids." That said, if providers working with another sort of therapy come away from reading this work with a useful way to articulate what it is that they do in a group that increases their effectiveness, we will be well pleased!

ACT Lends Itself to Dissemination

In chapter 1 we will examine relational frame theory (RFT) and the implications of what experts have learned about thinking and language. The result is a fully formed psychological model that accounts for both psychological suffering and psychological flexibility. ACT offers an approach that is not only evidence based but applicable to a wide range of presenting problems.

Because it is the ground-up, clinical derivative of what we have learned from basic applied science, we know not only *that* ACT works but also *why* it works and how we might then optimize the treatment. This is good stuff, especially if you are involved in training or supervising other mental health professionals. It is tremendously helpful in supervision to be able to articulate what it was that made a particular intervention effective (or not), and what might be a useful direction in which to head.

ACT Offers a Unifying Psychological Model

One result of working with an effective therapy is that providers can become fused with the idea that it is the "right" approach, and we have seen this in ACT therapists. There is a contradiction here. As we will discuss in chapter 1, ACT is based on functional contextualism, of which one implication is that constructs such as right or wrong, or better or worse, are just that: derived constructs. ACT is intensely pragmatic, focusing on what is workable in a given context. This certainly includes other therapeutic approaches that are beneficial to clients in some way. ACT is *a* way to assist clients, not *the* way.

Being contextually based means that ACT is not inherently in opposition to other ways of doing things. In fact, we make the case that many therapies incorporate the principles supported in ACT. We also point out that the core processes that are the specific focus of ACT are present in all behavior, which must include what is happening in other forms of therapy. That said, the objectives of ACT can directly contradict what some forms of therapy—most obviously, those aimed at eliminating symptoms or fixing thoughts—strive to achieve.

How to Use This Book

This book is intended to be used by therapists who have conducted group therapy but are new to the ACT model. We also believe that those who are familiar with the ACT model will benefit from learning how to apply the model to the group setting. Here are some suggestions:

1. Skip around. If you see topics that are quite familiar to you, it's okay to move on to the next section or chapter.

2. Look for what's missing from your knowledge base. There are many aspects to this book, from learning relational frame theory, to understanding the core ACT processes, to setting up ACT groups in different settings.

3. Drop into the group setting. We provide many example scenarios derived from our own experiences in groups and in supervising others. Our hope is that these will give you a real sense of what the dialogue in an ACT group looks like. You might find some surprises here if you are new to the model.

4. Approach what's new with scientific curiosity. It's easy to be dismissive of new approaches and want to stay rooted in what is familiar to you. See whether you can tip your heart and mind open to something new.

Structure of This Book and Online Accessories

This book is parsed into two main sections, part 1: Why ACT in Groups? and part 2: Applying ACT in a Group Setting. In part 1, chapter 1 provides a basic introduction to ACT. We discuss the philosophy of science and the theory (RFT) that produced the model, and how six fundamental behavioral processes fit into this framework. Throughout this book we stress that understanding the *why* guides every step of the *how* in ACT. So we take care to delineate how the principles that form the model directly apply to what we do in the therapy room. Chapters 2 and 3 extend this discussion, exploring the ways in which ACT can enhance the clinical opportunities available in group settings. Our hope is that interested readers will begin to see what this approach brings to the table.

Part 2 leads us through the application of ACT in a group setting, beginning with chapter 4, which provides a framework for getting started in ACT. We lay out the main objectives for an ACT group and a general strategy for meeting those objectives. This includes the various interventions that will be employed and what treatment planning (for a hypothetical group) might look like in this setting. We also examine certain tensions and challenges that arise from using ACT as a model as these come into play at the outset of therapy.

In chapters 5 through 10 we walk through an example group application of ACT, with each chapter focusing on a different core process. Each chapter includes specific objectives, key topics to cover, and example exercises and metaphors we have found to be effective in a group setting. Our example group has closed membership and has a clear start and end date. However, we recognize that this is just one of many possible clinical scenarios, and in chapter 11 we examine some important considerations to make when applying ACT to different group contexts.

In an effort to stay consistent with our emphasis on operating from the process level with ACT, we deliberately chose to organize part 2 by the core processes and skills being addressed rather than by session, so as not to suggest that the therapist's choices about how to proceed in session were driven by the session number.

And, we have a bonus for you! There is supplementary content for our book available at http://www.newharbinger.com/23994. Here you will find a "Supplemental Exercises" document containing additional exercises for use in your groups along with commentary and further insights about conducting ACT in groups. Additionally, you may download handouts as well as "Furthering Your ACT Skills," which contains numerous resources to help you learn more about ACT and hone your skills. We invite you to use these valuable supplemental resources.

Why We Wrote This Book

We started this book with the pronouncement that ACT makes a significant contribution to group treatment, and a growing body of data supports our case. ACT groups are now used throughout the world for difficulties as diverse as substance abuse, post-traumatic stress disorder (PTSD), anxiety, depression, anger, smoking cessation, and work stress. It is used with children, at-risk youth, adults, the elderly, and people with disabilities. From this work, several studies examining ACT as a group intervention have emerged. The results are quite promising, indicating that ACT in groups has compared well to other popular forms of group treatment. (We refer interested readers to the Association for Contextual Behavioral Science [ACBS] website, https://www.contextualscience.org.)

The main reason we wished to write this book is that we both have directly experienced the power of ACT as a group treatment. We are convinced not only that ACT can be done skillfully in groups of all kinds, but that it can uniquely synergize therapeutic healing in a group context.

We find it great fun to chew on this stuff. But perhaps that doesn't speak to the awe we feel when we witness how participation in an ACT group can change a person's life. We are also grateful for the opportunity to offer what we've learned to others interested in applying ACT in groups. We promise to do our best to pass on what we have learned about this compelling and powerful therapy.

PART 1

WHY ACT IN GROUPS?

CHAPTER 1

An Introduction to ACT

We have stated our belief that ACT can dramatically increase the effectiveness of group therapy, and we will make the case further in chapters 2 and 3. This chapter is intended as an introduction to ACT. For those who are unfamiliar with ACT, this chapter will give you a grounding in the history, theory, and practice of ACT, and the most important assumptions and concepts that characterize the model. (If you're already familiar with ACT's theoretical foundations, its model of psychopathology, and its six core processes, feel free to skip this chapter and go straight to chapter 2.)

Contextual Behavioral Science: Mapping Research to Real Life

When it comes to understanding human behavior, there is a natural gap between the research lab and our everyday lives. Our species has been in the business of being human for a while now—we certainly haven't waited for scientific explanations before figuring out ways to improve our lot! It makes sense that over time humans would develop techniques geared to alleviate suffering and that some of those practices would have staying power. For example, seeking and receiving support from others—an important aspect of both individual and group therapy—is one of the earliest ways we found to help ourselves, necessary in fact to our basic survival. It remains one of the most important factors in well-being today, believed to be a mitigating factor in both psychological and physical health. Similarly, the practices of mindfulness meditation and active acceptance have been around a long time, especially in some parts of the world, and remain relevant today. But only recently have we begun to fully appreciate what such techniques can offer in medical and therapeutic settings, the workplace, educational systems, and other domains.

A key contribution of ACT, or more specifically of relational frame theory (RFT; Hayes, Strosahl, & Wilson, 1999), upon which ACT is based, is that it helps us understand *why* practices like these are helpful. It has narrowed the gap between what simple experience tells us and our understanding of the actual processes involved. Further, developing the science has served to not only clarify but extend what we know about being human. We begin to understand how it is that we humans can become so stuck. We also begin to see why certain approaches to alleviate suffering are ineffective, and what a more workable approach might entail.

One way to think about RFT is that it illuminates the varying ways in which clients present in therapy and in their lives. More specifically, it illuminates fundamental behaviors that we all have in common that both help and hinder us to varying degrees. Learning to recognize these can be quite useful, not only as a way to understand the struggle, but also as a way to focus the therapy and move things forward. While ACT is designed to specifically target the key processes highlighted in RFT, we believe that having some familiarity with them would prove helpful to any therapist.

The Study of Thinking: It's About Language

It took a while for behavioral scientists to tackle one of the most fundamental aspects of being human—thinking, that is. Although clinicians and researchers from varying theoretical orientations generally have agreed that thoughts play a major role in our experience, the behavior of thinking itself is not easily examined. We have come to learn, however, that even this covert phenomenon can be studied using basic applied research methodologies. Over the past two decades, this area of inquiry, now known as contextual behavioral science, has continued to develop and has led to some pretty important discoveries about what it is to be human.

Most essentially, research has demonstrated a great deal about the role the ability to develop language plays in the human experience. The study of thinking necessarily involves the study of language acquisition (you need words to have thoughts), and as scientists learned more about how we develop language, they began to identify particular abilities that appear to be uniquely human. These abilities allow us to create a verbal virtual reality (the world of our thoughts) that comes to exert a great deal of influence in our lives. One reason for this is that we actually aren't aware that languaging is a behavior and thoughts are the result. We relate to this product (our thoughts) as representing "truth," which can be very problematic. We see the manifestations of this everywhere, certainly in group therapy and in our daily lives as well. If you have ever been frustrated because you repeatedly do something that costs you, if you know of someone who just can't see what a great person she is, or if someone you care about can't get past something even though it is ruining his life—languaging offers both an explanation and a direction in which to head.

Relational Frame Theory: How It Works

One of the key elements in developing language is being able to infer or relate things based on something other than simple physical characteristics. As an example, let's compare a dog and a human. A dog, like a toddler, can learn to associate sounds with particular objects based on their physical characteristics. For example, the dog can learn that the long, skinny, wooden object she loves to chase after is a "stick." Her owner could command, "Stick!" and the dog would run around, nose to the ground, looking for something with those physical characteristics.

Now let's take a child. As a toddler, a child will learn to relate things in this same way, but unlike the dog, he will also learn something about the relation itself. Using the above example, like the dog, the child registers the physical properties of the object and learns that the long, skinny, wooden object is the same as the spoken word "stick." However, the child will also come to learn the meaning of the relation: *same as*. It is this ability that will allow the child to associate various other objects based on the *same as* relation alone. As he develops, he will eventually be able to learn, for example, that squiggles on a piece of paper (i.e., writing) are the *same as* the spoken word "stick." The child also has the ability to infer an additional relation between things: that if those squiggles are the same as the *spoken word* "stick," those squiggles must then also be the same as the actual *object* (i.e., the stick itself). We have exceeded the dog's capabilities here. Note that the child can also be told to throw a knotted rope "like a stick" and proceed to make the rope function like a stick even though there is little physical similarity between the two.

This ability to understand and derive relations between things allows human beings to link anything together, regardless of physical properties—indeed, even if what is being linked does not physically exist. For example, the child will likely learn somewhere along the line that being physically injured results in pain, and that being injured is therefore something to be avoided. Because of his ability to understand and derive relations, he will also come to learn that a concept termed "dangerous" is the *same as* something that injures, so that "dangerous" is *automatically* linked to something that causes physical pain and should therefore be avoided. The parent can call out, "Careful with that stick—it's dangerous!" (the stick is the *same as* dangerous), and that statement will rapidly be connected to all those previously derived relations. It will now convey significant meaning, even though a thing called "dangerous" does not actually exist in the physical sense, and the child has never experienced being hurt by a stick. Useful stuff!

However, it is this same ability to derive relations between anything that can lead us to produce the thought *I am a failure* and then relate to that thought as though failure physically exists within us. This linking ability becomes so automatic that we miss it. We miss that we are actively linking our selfhood to a concept and then relating to what we have created as though we are that product. We think, *I am a failure* as opposed to *I am linking these ideas together and the result is the thought that I am a failure.*

We begin to see now how this useful languaging ability can also be a torment. To explore a bit further, consider another of the many types of relations we learn when we acquire language: that of *comparison*. Not only do we learn to compare two objects and discern which one is "bigger," for example, but the comparative relations themselves take on meaning. *Bigger than, smaller than, more than, less than, better than, worse than*—through language acquisition these terms come to have their own meaning even though they do not exist in the physical world. That child will come to learn the meaning of an evaluative construct such as "worst" (when something called "worst" doesn't physically exist), and that being called the "worst hitter" on his baseball team is therefore not a good thing. Notice how this will entail an emotional component as well. That is, "worst hitter" is not just a mental concept. Previous learning around bad/worst involved a subjective experience (e.g., feelings of shame) that is also transferred as the link between "worst" and "hitter" is made. Being called the "worst hitter" will bring that prior emotional response—possibly even unpleasant physical sensations—into the present. Before the child developed language, however, "You are the worst hitter" would simply have been heard as a bunch of sounds.

In this way, languaging intrudes upon the present and even the future. Things that are not a part of our physical present persist in the world of our thoughts. They impact how we experience the physical world and influence our behavior. Telling a dog he is the "worst retriever" means nothing to the dog, who continues to enjoy fetching the stick for as long as she is rewarded for doing so (i.e., her owner throwing the stick). The boy, however, could give up on baseball for good, regardless of what occurs in his actual environment. He could proceed to have a good hit, for example, but continue to dwell on what it means to be the worst hitter on his team. In fact, because we are continually linking things together ("hitter" is linked to baseball, baseball is linked to sports, and so forth), being called the "worst hitter" could result in the boy avoiding sports activities the rest of his life. He has established a "relational network" around the idea of sports that he now carries with him through time.

We mentioned earlier that clarity into these language processes sheds light on how we humans can get stuck, as we saw in the above example. We are constantly deriving relations between things, and it is not something we can stop. The result is that constantly streaming ticker tape of thoughts we all experience. It is quite seductive. It tends to get our full attention. So not only do we miss the fact that we are the ones producing all this and take our thoughts literally, we lose contact with our actual environment. We become fused with whatever is running on that cognitive ticker tape, living in that verbal virtual reality even if it costs us dearly. A thought such as *I'm not confident enough to apply for that job* is purely language based (a thing called "confidence" is not physically missing in the person). Nonetheless, it can override what our actual experience might tell us. We miss, for example, the opportunity to learn that we can apply for a job without the feeling of confidence—or that we can survive the discomfort of not feeling confident. In this way we lose sight of what is going on in our actual lives and behave in ways that reinforce what's in our heads.

Here we see how easy it is for humans to continue doing things that are actually problematic for them. In essence, the verbal virtual reality comes to be *the* reality, outweighing information that is available in the physical environment. The group member who is invested in being right, for example, is likely fused with verbal rules that have been derived over time. He could have made the link somewhere along the line that being "wrong" was the same as being "stupid," which was the same as being "unacceptable" (notice that things called "wrong," "stupid," and "unacceptable" don't actually exist in the physical world). Perhaps he has formed a bunch of associations around what it means to feel vulnerable. Regardless, he produces *and buys* those rules that have been relationally derived, and then he behaves accordingly. Those rules outweigh what is happening around him, including the consequences of his behavior. If his attention wasn't with the rules, for instance, he might have the opportunity to learn from his environment that being wrong is in fact survivable, or that his interactions with others improve when he allows himself to be wrong.

What we are exploring here are fundamental principles of languaging, which means they apply to us all. Just as a client is caught up in a relational network that can include such thoughts as *I am broken because of my trauma*, *No one can be trusted*, and *My life is over*, we all are fused with any number of thoughts during the course of a typical day: *I'm just not motivated enough to go to the gym. That guy is such a jerk! I'm never going to finish this.* Note that this unavoidable phenomenon is not restricted to "negative" thoughts. *I always honor my commitments* is an example of the same languaging ability—just one that tends to serve a more workable purpose in our lives.

Before wrapping up our brief foray into RFT, we'd like to point to another implication of what we have learned about the role of language. We can see now why it doesn't work so well to try to get clients (or our friends, our family, or ourselves) to get rid of difficult thoughts and feelings. The deriving of relations has occurred (and is occurring); the network has been developed (and is developing); we can't just will our way into that network and wipe out a troubling element here or there. Nor does adding new stuff (e.g., a more "positive" point of view) somehow erase or override what is already there. If you have ever tried to get someone with very low self-esteem to view himself differently, you have run into this difficulty. As another example, individuals with PTSD know all too well how futile it is to try to eliminate a memory. How many times have *you* thought you were "over" something only to discover (when the right contextual cue came along) that you weren't over it at all? So aligning with our clients in their endeavor to eradicate certain thoughts or memories just adds to the existing verbal network, which will now include ideas such as *I must not be doing this right*, *This just proves how messed up I am*, *I should be over this by now*, or *I'm never going to be normal.*

Up to now, we have been exploring the role that languaging plays in our lives, including how this ability can lead to great suffering. Since losing ourselves in our thoughts and relating to them in a very literal way can be problematic, it follows that learning how to see thoughts for what they actually are—to "de-literalize" them—would prove helpful. If one cost of being lost in a verbal virtual reality is awareness of our physical environment and how our behavior actually functions (i.e., the actual vs.

imagined consequences to what we do or don't do), then learning to be present and tracking what is actually going on might help us get unstuck. And since we have this powerful ability to construct a verbal virtual reality that we carry with us through time, might it be possible to create verbal links that serve to enhance our lives? These are some of the implications and questions that gave rise to ACT, and we will turn now to an exploration of this treatment approach.

What Is ACT?

ACT was first presented as a treatment in 1999. As we discussed, however, this followed twenty-some years of basic applied research into human cognition and language acquisition. We have briefly summarized some of the key findings and implications of this effort, but there are excellent resources available that provide much more thorough accountings. (See, for example, the seminal text *Acceptance and Commitment Therapy: The Process and Practice of Mindful Change* by Hayes, Strosahl, and Wilson [2011].) We will now point out a couple of things about the philosophical and theoretical underpinnings of ACT that influence the intervention in important ways.

Contextualism and Behaviorism: The Roots and Heart of ACT

The approach to human behavior seen in ACT is rooted in *functional contextualism*, a philosophy of science that holds that everything exists and occurs within a context. Since we can't separate anything out from the context in which it occurs, we can't really get at "truth," because that will always be influenced by the current context. The focus of functional contextualism, therefore, is highly pragmatic: "What's true is what works" (Hayes et al., 2011, p. 33). This idea is also at the heart of *radical behaviorism*, a psychological approach that assumes all behavior has a function. To understand a behavior's function, we must examine the context in which it occurs (what comes before and after).

We see the respective influences of these schools of thought in ACT's pragmatic treatment approach. Rather than operate from the position that certain behaviors or diagnoses are inherently bad or abnormal (because that sort of "truth" can't be proven), the focus is on *workability*. We ask: how is the behavior actually functioning in the client's life? Whether or not a behavior is "workable" or not depends on its consequences. A brief example will better illustrate this key distinction:

Consider an individual who is "withdrawn." Before continuing, notice what comes up in your own mind even as you read that sentence. Because of those vast relational networks you've developed, it is likely this imagined individual was quickly linked to whatever associations you have around the concept of being withdrawn. In fact, we don't yet know what being withdrawn means to this individual. To understand this, we need to discover how being withdrawn is actually functioning for this person at a given point in time. We can imagine a scenario where responding in a withdrawn manner is costly (e.g., a man whose withdrawn behavior at work cost him a promotion) and one in which it appears to work well (e.g., a woman recovering from an illness who seeks quiet and rest). Notice that as you assess these two scenarios, part of what you are taking into consideration is consequences. That is, because the man's withdrawing behavior resulted in not being promoted, it seems his behavior was not too workable for him. Because quiet and rest are typically viewed as positive consequences (thanks to the relations we've previously derived, by the way), the woman's choice to withdraw might be deemed a workable decision. However, imagine that we learned that the man had no interest in the job promotion and had purposefully behaved in a way that would ensure he remained in his current position. In this case, his behavior was successful and workable in his view. Similarly, the woman recovering from illness might find that her self-enforced solitude led to feeling lonely and depressed. Or imagine that she suddenly worsened to the point of being critically ill, and per her instructions, no one stopped by or called to check up on her!

We are naturally engaging in what we would more formally call a *functional assessment*. We are examining and developing a hypothesis about the behavior's context, specifically what came before the behavior, or the antecedent (not wanting a promotion, an illness and fatigue), and what followed, or the consequences. Workability is then based on this assessment, not on a determination that withdrawn behavior is inherently wrong or bad.

What is probably not apparent in this rather technical discussion about the underpinnings of ACT is that the therapy has great "heart." ACT sessions are typically deeply compassionate. Clients are not viewed as abnormal, sick, or broken in some way. The stuff they do, even if very problematic in their lives, is seen as just that—unworkable behavior—rather than evidence of some sort of pathology within them. We start with the assumption that clients are whole and acceptable as they are. There are three main reasons for this: (1) "abnormal" or "deficient" and the like can't be empirically established as being "true" (everything is influenced by context and cannot be separated out from that context); (2) we understand that such concepts are the products of languaging anyway; and (3) as the principles forming the ACT model apply to us all, there is a leveling of the playing field between therapist and client that brings humbleness to the approach. In understanding that we all deal with these things to varying degrees, we contact deep compassion and respect for the struggle of being human.

Psychological Flexibility and the Six Core Processes of ACT

So what is our actual objective in ACT? As described by Hayes, Strosahl, and Wilson (2011), *psychological flexibility* is our goal. "Psychological flexibility can be defined as contacting the present moment as a conscious human being, fully and without needless defense—as it is and not what it says it is—and persisting with or changing behavior in the service of chosen values" (pp. 96–97). In short, we aim to use the information gained from studying language and cognition to help clients get unstuck and vitally engaged in their lives.

As we explore the following processes targeted in ACT, it is important to understand that these abilities are highly interrelated. That is, they reflect particular aspects of psychological flexibility, but while distinct, they do not actually stand alone. Ability in one core process both reflects and influences ability in another. It is also important to remember that because psychological flexibility is on a continuum, each of the involved processes is also on a continuum. Just as strengths in these areas define psychological flexibility, deficits represent the varying ways in which clients can be stuck. Let's take a look at the six core processes in detail:

CONTACTING THE PRESENT

We've mentioned how once language comes along we are pulled into the world of our thoughts, losing contact with important aspects of our actual lives. As we discussed, one cost is opportunities to experience and learn from a reality beyond that offered by our minds. There is another cost. While being present might sometimes (even often) entail contacting painful thoughts and feelings, this is also where "the good stuff" lives. Vitality, joy, authentic connection…these are present-moment experiences that we miss when we are stuck in our heads. This is why one of the core abilities fostered in ACT is the ability to contact the present moment as it unfolds. As viewed in ACT, being present as a destination or stable state is not the goal (even if that were possible). Rather, in ACT we aim to develop the ability to flexibly bring our attention to various aspects of our current experience. That might be attending to our breathing, our feelings, our actions, our thoughts, what we see, what we sense, and so on.

WILLINGNESS/ACCEPTANCE

Willingness, also referred to as *acceptance*, is defined in ACT as the ability to experience the present without engaging in some sort of control or change strategy, in other words trying to escape, alter, or ignore the thoughts, feelings, and bodily sensations present at any given moment. (Though we also use the term "acceptance" in this book, we typically use "willingness" when wanting to emphasize the active nature of this process). Not only are we hardwired to seek physiological homeostasis, but our relationship with language has resulted in clear ideas around what is, and is not, okay to experience internally. We learn to evaluate our thoughts and feelings as good or bad, and then we buy those evaluations as being literally true (that verbal virtual reality again). For example, somewhere along the line, like us, you probably learned that it is not okay to feel unhappy. We didn't come into the world thinking that way, nor is it likely that the cow standing in a field in the rain is thinking, *This is unacceptable*. However, for verbal beings these sorts of "shoulds" and similar rules are developed as we acquire language. We then go to great effort to avoid experiences we have deemed to be unacceptable.

In essence, not only does languaging dispose us to lose contact with what is happening in our physical lives, but the relational network we develop leads us to believe that (a) there are certain internal experiences we should be having and those we should not be having, and (b) we need to get out of unwanted experiences somehow. Our subsequent efforts to control or avoid cost us opportunities to learn otherwise. In fact, according to these sorts of rules, the fact that we are not succeeding at eliminating discomfort is simply further evidence that something is wrong and that we just need to work harder.

DEFUSION

Arising directly from our understanding of language processes, a key target in ACT is helping clients learn to de-literalize their thoughts. We call this the ability to *defuse* from thoughts, to see them for what they are (i.e., something we behaviorally produce) as opposed to buying them as "truth." So when a client has the thought *I am a failure*, we hope to help him shift from holding that thought as being literally true (being fused with the thought) to thinking, *I am having that thought again about being a failure* (defusing from the thought). This entails the ability to look *at* a thought rather than simply *from* a thought.

This represents a profound shift in perspective. One of the more significant ramifications of being fused with thoughts is the constraints this places on our behavior. We buy the rules in our head, such as *I'm too shy to speak in public* or *I'm not acceptable with this trauma*, and act accordingly. When we learn to see thoughts as thoughts, we have greater awareness of the behavioral choices that are actually before us. It's sort of like, *I have the thought… So now what?* If thoughts don't represent literal truth, if we don't have to do what our minds tell us, what then?

We begin to see how these processes are indeed interrelated. Being able to notice and defuse from thoughts requires *getting present*. At the same time, being in touch with the present can certainly include noticing (looking at, not just from) our thoughts. Contacting the present sets the stage for willingness, while willingness enables us to be present. Similarly, our next core process is reflected in the above processes while serving to extend them even further.

SELF-AS-CONTEXT

This is a key process in ACT, and yet it is often one of the hardest to understand and work with effectively. Although *self-as-context* is an ability we aim to foster, we also examine two other ways of experiencing the self in ACT. These are (1) the conceptualized self, and (2) self-as-process. As we work through these, we will see again that while each one points to a particular aspect of self-experience, each influences the other (and other core ACT processes as well).

The conceptualized self. Earlier in this chapter we examined how acquiring language involves the key ability to link things together based on relations such as *same as* or *more/less than*. We also mentioned that we learn to apply other types of relations as well (the term we use for this overall ability is *relational framing*). A full discussion of relational framing would be a book unto itself, and fortunately there are already excellent texts that do the job well. (See, for example, *Learning RFT* [Torneke, 2010] and *The Self and Perspective Taking* [McHugh & Stewart, 2012]). For now, we will simply say that when it comes to our own selves, we use certain types of relations to build our very identity. It is not until we learn language that we learn to identify that constant locus of perspective moving through time as being the "I," for example. Via relational framing we come to define ourselves based on physical characteristics and learned labels (e.g., "I am Sarah"; "I am a girl"). With that ability comes the ability to also link evaluations and categorizations to that "I" (e.g., "I am smart"; "I am clumsy"). Eventually we come to derive an entire identity—a conceptualized self—made up of these sorts of descriptions, categorizations, and evaluations.

Having conceptualized selves is not problematic per se. In fact, this ability is key to functioning in our world. Imagine attempting to move through our lives without knowing our names, our gender, our profession, our qualifications, and so forth. However, because we become fused with the product and lose the process, we treat our conceptualized selves as literal truths, at times at great cost. A client raised in an abusive, neglectful environment will have developed an identity that could well include such ideas as *Something's wrong with me*, *I'm not enough*, and *I'm shameful*, and then hold these as literally true—as though "shameful" and the like could be physically found within him. This in turn influences how the client experiences himself and others and also the behavioral choices he makes throughout his life. As another example, someone could have such a rigid attachment to being "smart" that she will not tolerate any experience that would suggest otherwise (e.g., failing at something new). As discussed previously, we now understand how it is that clients can have intractable notions of themselves despite others' attempts to persuade them otherwise. That is, once connected, these things can't be unconnected. However, we can help clients to see their conceptualized selves for what they are (constructed identities) and to hold these in a less rigid, more workable way.

Self-as-process. This refers to the ability to notice the thoughts, feelings, and sensations we are experiencing at a given point in time. Examples are noticing that your heart is pounding and that your palms are sweaty, or noticing that you are experiencing the feeling of fear and are having thoughts such as *I have to get out of here*. Getting present and experiencing defusion come into play with self-as-process; we need to be present to our experience to notice it, and we need to be able to look at our thoughts a bit to pull them out and articulate them as something we experienced.

Building the ability to experience self-as-process is an important target in ACT, and we promote it via explicit discussion, use of metaphors, and experiential exercises. We also promote it by intentional language use throughout the session. That is, when working with our clients, we use—and encourage them to use—words that highlight the process aspect of experience. "I *am having* the thought that something terrible is going to happen," "I *am experiencing* a rapid heartbeat," and "I *am having* that feeling of dread again" all point to such internal processes as phenomena of the moment.

Self-as-context. In assisting clients to experience self-as-process, we pave the way for them to experience self-as-context. By this we mean not only recognizing thoughts, feelings, and sensations as they occur, but also bringing awareness to who's doing all the noticing. Clients are guided to "notice the Noticer"—that constant locus of perspective that has been there through time and through experience, a perspective that is thus both stable and larger than the thoughts, feelings, and sensations of the moment. Self-as-context is awareness of that locus of perspective as both distinct from, and including, those inner experiences.

In some ACT texts this is described as the *transcendent self*, and this sort of self-experience can indeed have a transcendent, even spiritual, quality. In recognizing the distinction between Experiencer and experiences (meaning thoughts, feelings, and sensations), we are freed from having to battle those experiences (while we continue to experience them). Experiencing self-as-context can have a timeless, boundary-less quality that engenders a sense of connection with the world and to life itself.

That said, our objective in ACT remains a pragmatic one. We hope to help clients access these varying ways of experiencing the self so that they can respond to life in a more flexible, workable, and ultimately vital way. We emphasize that all these ways of self-experiencing are behavioral processes—abilities that people demonstrate to varying degrees at any point in time.

VALUES

Earlier we made the point that defusing from thoughts can lead to a sort of "What next" experience. That is, if thoughts and feelings aren't in charge and if we don't actually have to fix or get rid of them, on what do we base our behavior? We arrive at values as a guide—not as a "should," but more because we can. There is inherent meaning found in making choices according to deeply held values. We help clients identify what they care about and how they want to be moving through the world. In this way we intentionally use the same language processes that can get clients stuck to help them actually live the way they want to be living.

For example, if a client is in pain because he has been a "bad dad," it follows he has a notion of what being a good dad would entail. We can (via languaging and relational framing) help him articulate what being a good dad looks like for him and identify specific behaviors that take him in that valued direction. Earlier we talked about how we tend to live in a verbal virtual reality at the cost of being aware of our actual environment. In being fused with imagined or anticipated consequences of our behavior, for example, we miss learning about actual consequences. By identifying values and establishing a clear link between behavioral choices and living those values, we help clients track whether their actions are taking them closer to, or further away from, how they want to be living. This in turn helps them access the intrinsic rewards available in making value-driven choices.

COMMITTED ACTION

The process that is the most easily explained is also the most important. That is, all of the core process work means little if it doesn't translate into clients living their lives vitally and well. In ACT we want clients to "get moving with their feet." We make the point that whether it be an inch or a mile, moving toward values is moving toward values. The intention is that the reinforcing qualities of value-driven action will lead to an ever-expanding pattern of behavior that is *open*, *centered*, and *engaged*.

Doing ACT in Groups

So how does one bring this complex of interlocking concepts and processes into a group therapeutic setting? In part 2, we will walk you through how to apply ACT in one type of group setting, and we will discuss some clinical implications of applying the therapy in other types of groups in chapter 11. Regardless of the particular strategy for moving through the therapy, the focus is on furthering the six core processes. This is a key point because it is easy to treat the content of ACT—the various exercises, topics, and metaphors—as being the therapy. This is a common misstep. In ACT, discussion topics, exercises, metaphors, and simple conversation are ways to flush out and build ability with the core processes. The therapy is about the processes, not all the content. This means there will be many ways to "do ACT" so long as those core processes are being advanced.

In sum, we seek to assess clients' abilities with the core processes and determine how these play out in their lives. Deficits tend to manifest as being stuck: stuck in thoughts, stuck in unworkable behaviors, stuck in lives that lack vitality and meaning. The therapy is designed to flush out these processes and then provide ways to help build these six core behavioral abilities.

Summary

Our intention with this chapter was to provide readers with a sense of ACT—the research that led to it, the theoretical foundations, and the essence of what this therapy is all about. We have not taken a "beginner's approach," however. That is, some applied texts spend less time on the theory behind ACT and focus more on the *how* of ACT. (Don't worry; we will get to that, too.) There is a real benefit to making the therapy as accessible and approachable as possible; indeed, the growth seen in the clinical application of ACT is in large part owed to these efforts. However, we also have seen that when therapists lack the *why* of ACT, it can be harder to actually do the therapy and certainly easier to step off the model.

We chose to go straight to the principles in ACT, with the hope that you will begin to see both their import and how they manifest in the therapy room. As we work through the *how* of ACT in part 2, we will take a practical, clinician-friendly approach while also highlighting how what we do reflects fidelity to these principles. In the end, our hope is that you will be able to recognize these, articulate their function, and enable those with whom you work to move toward being more psychologically flexible in their lives.

CHAPTER 2

The Power of ACT in Groups

One of the greatest challenges in learning to conduct ACT effectively is learning to view the therapy through an "ACT lens": to translate what you are observing and experiencing to the model's core processes. Once it's familiar, however, there is a beautiful simplicity to this approach. The processes represent fundamental principles of human behavior, crossing diagnoses, symptoms, and backgrounds. The commonality of these processes provides an always-accessible clinical guideline. As our facility with the processes builds, we become increasingly able to recognize how they manifest—in our clients' lives, in the therapy group, and in ourselves as well. We also have a unifying clinical goal. That is, we seek to further the psychological flexibility of all members by building their abilities with the core processes. This enables them, regardless of their differences, to respond to whatever life is handing them in a more workable and vital way. This singular guide is extremely helpful in the extra-dynamic context of groups.

Let's take a moment and imagine a therapy group. It doesn't really matter what kind; take whatever comes to mind. Membership could be based on a common difficulty (e.g., grief, domestic violence), diagnosis (e.g., PTSD, depression), or setting (e.g., outpatient center, inpatient hospital). Regardless of these factors, participants bring their individual histories and ways of approaching life to the group. This means that one member might dominate the sessions, while another might refuse to take any risks. One might laugh inappropriately whenever things get a little emotional; another might pit himself against the therapist and engage in debate at any opportunity. Another member might present as apathetic throughout, seeming to care about nothing, while another might expend great effort trying to please, and so on. What these group members likely have in common is that something isn't working in their lives. What they also have in common is that the way they respond to their life experience has played a part in this, just as it is playing a role in the therapy room.

We can imagine that some of these members will carry clinical diagnoses of some sort, and we know they will all have histories that play a part in how they are experiencing and engaging with the world. Understanding that they are all somewhere along the continuum of psychological flexibility provides a common thread. Despite their differences, each demonstrates varying ability with the core processes of contacting and being willing to experience the present, defusing from thoughts, experiencing self-as-context, and engaging in life according to identified values. Regardless of their disparate histories or symptoms, regardless of the differences in what they are searching for or facing, furthering these core abilities will enable them to hold their experiences in a more useful way and move forward in their lives.

Let's look again at our hypothetical group. The member who dominates the session may be highly fused with what his mind is telling him, so stuck in his "stories" that he is not present to other members or how his behavior negatively impacts the group. He may be unwilling to experience the feelings of tension or anxiety that are there when he's not so busy talking. The member who holds back from participating may be fused with what sharing guarded details about herself might mean and may be unwilling to experience the vulnerability of opening up. She may believe that others will find her unacceptable if they really get to know her. In other words, she is rigidly attached to a conceptualized self. The group member who laughs inappropriately may be unwilling to experience intense emotion and fused with the notion that feeling uncomfortable is not okay.

The member who spends the sessions debating with the therapist could be fused with his thoughts and acting in the service of verbal rules despite the interpersonal costs (which could also represent unwillingness and rigid attachment to a conceptualized self). Or perhaps the experience of being right simply feels good, and the issue is more that the member is pursuing that experience rather than living his values around developing good relationships.

Let's play this out some more: The apathetic member might be stuck in unwillingness ("not caring" as a way to avoid) or fusion ("There's no point"). He may have lost contact with the sorts of things that provided a sense of meaning and vitality in his life (i.e., lack of identified values and committed action). The member trying so hard to please could believe that her value comes from others (i.e., fusion, attachment to a conceptualized self, unwillingness to displease others or experience rejection).

We could extend this discussion and imagine ways in which these behaviors show up in each member's life outside of session. The point is that despite very different presentations, these core abilities are in play. It follows, then, that building these abilities—enhancing psychological flexibility—would prove helpful. Regardless of history or life situation, being able to respond to what life is handing out in a way that is open (willing and defused), centered (present and aware of self-as-context), and engaged (values and committed action) stands a good chance of making a meaningful difference for each group member.

ACT Clarifies Treatment Targets

You have likely already perceived how the commonality of these processes is useful in and of itself. If you are anything like us, there have been many times when you've been completely flummoxed in a group therapy session. Often in groups there is simply a ton going on and any number of possible directions in which to head. And then there are those sessions when an uncomfortable, flat silence seems to be the order of the day. What in the heck do you do with that? What we have found is that when we learn to look for how things are functioning, for the process rather than the content, we find that, indeed, the core ACT processes are at work. Identifying these processes helps us refrain from being reactive and instead remain intentional with our intervention. We better understand how increasing these key abilities leads to more workable ways of being in the group and in life more broadly. We are better able to avoid getting stuck in something unproductive and focus in on what might help members progress. We will explore ways to maximize this benefit of using ACT in chapter 3.

ACT Sharpens Clinical Decision Making

This naturally follows from the points just made. That is, when you learn to recognize the processes at work in a given situation, you are provided with ideas as to how you might productively proceed. Imagine, for example, that a group member just expressed a very "negative" (we would call it costly, depending on the context) view of himself as being "toxic." In this moment you might recognize he is fused with this thought. He is buying it as being literally true—as if a thing called toxic is physically in him. This statement also suggests an inability to experience self-as-context. The group member does not seem to be in touch with the distinction between Thinker and thought, nor does he understand that he is larger than the thoughts and feelings of the moment.

And there is likely more. For example, if he were less in his head and more present to the group, he might be tracking that others are not reacting to him as though he is toxic. (Even if they *are* turned off by his behavior, it's unlikely they're lying poisoned and prostrate on the ground!) It is possible that avoidance is at work; perhaps it is more comfortable for him to remain with his thoughts about being toxic than risk being actually rejected.

This may seem like a lot of possible processes going on. The thing is, it will always be the same core processes, in contrast to the unlimited content members can potentially introduce in a group session. Further, the same processes revealed in the one member's "toxic" comment will be present in the behaviors of the other group members as well. Following this comment, for example, another member of the group might tune out, manifesting (hypothetically, we must remember) avoidance, fusion, and not being present. Another member might immediately try to rescue her peer, demonstrating unwillingness to experience what she feels when someone expresses such a belief and fusion with the notion that such thoughts must be corrected. When we learn to look at all this behavior through an ACT lens, we find common processes that can be highlighted and worked on to the benefit of each group member.

It is important to remember that these abilities are on a continuum and therefore account not just for deficits but for strengths as well. For example, imagine that following the "toxic" remark, a different group member jumped immediately into something going on with his own life (fusion, not being present, perhaps avoidance). However, he quickly caught himself (contacting the present moment, self-as-process, defusion), then apologized and asked his peer to continue with what he had been saying (values and committed action). In this way, learning to recognize the processes as they arise in session also helps you point out and reinforce members' positive moves.

ACT Increases Clinical Coherence and Consistency

If you ever want to conduct an interesting experiment, record one or two of your therapy sessions and then check to see whether the messages you sent were entirely consistent. This can be surprisingly difficult to achieve! For example, you might find that at one point you encourage your client to experience his feelings, and in another you work to make distressing feelings go away. You might provide evidence that the client is capable, and in the next imply that she is someone who needs your more expert help. You might explain why a thought does not actually cause a behavior, and then reveal an expectation that the client's behavior should automatically change now that he gets your point. In our experience, the opportunity to inadvertently send mixed messages is compounded in a group. Not only is there simply more going on, but you, as therapist, have varying reactions to each member of the group. You will be dealing with your own "shoulds" (due to those derived relations), which can make it challenging to maintain a consistent stance toward everyone in the group. You might be pulled to "protect" a certain member, for example, while hooked into debating with another. Additionally, you are not just working at the individual level, but at the group level as well. So you could earnestly be helping one member to contact her feelings while at the same time aligning in a group effort to avoid something that is happening in the room. The possibilities are endless.

The fact that all group members (including you) are somewhere along the continuum of psychological flexibility provides a mainstay for the session. When you are clear about the abilities that further psychological flexibility, you are better able to support them. You understand, for example, why we aim for altering how thoughts function for our clients rather than trying to eliminate them. This, in turn, suggests how you might work with all thoughts, regardless of their form. This is key given there's no limit to what clients can introduce in session. Similarly, you understand that being able to experience the present moment without defending or controlling is a skill to be developed by the group, which helps you refrain from engaging in those sorts of maneuvers yourself.

ACT Maximizes the Change Mechanisms of Groups

When done well, ACT magnifies therapeutic change mechanisms inherent in group work. Developed as the clinical response to an increased understanding of the origins of human suffering, the model articulates the processes that can keep humans stuck, and how those same processes can be used to alleviate suffering. This directly translates to the therapy room.

ACT Optimizes the Therapeutic Relationship

The importance of the therapeutic alliance in treatment effectiveness has been well-documented. Therapist qualities shown to enhance the therapist-client relationship are not only supported in ACT, but form the means by which the therapy is advanced. By being compassionately present, centered, and fully engaged, therapists provide a context that invites clients to do the same.

One of the fundamental aspects of the therapeutic relationship in ACT has already been mentioned: that therapists are as human as their clients. They too struggle with languaging and all it entails; they too experience being stuck in various ways. At any point in time, therapists are somewhere along the continuum of psychological flexibility and have the opportunity to make choices that take them closer to, or further away from, their values.

There is more. Remember that ACT is based upon RFT and what we have learned about our relationship with language. Being fused with, and blindly following, verbal rules around "being the expert" and "needing to look competent" is just that—fusion with verbal rules. In that stance there is little awareness of how our behavior is affecting the client and the therapy overall. When these sorts of thoughts, evaluations, and inclinations show up, as they are sure to do, the ACT therapist simply notices them rather than working not to have them, or operating from (fusing with) them. In so doing, she is contacting the present and noticing what is going on (which requires willingness, self-as-process, and defusion). She might choose to articulate her experience in the service of being consistent with the therapy and to model for the client—a generous example of all of the above combined with values and committed action. In short, the therapist is actively and intentionally working on (a) being psychologically flexible herself, (b) building a psychologically flexible therapeutic alliance, and (c) developing psychological flexibility in her client.

It can be a shock for therapists new to ACT to approach the therapy in this way. What they find, however, is that rather than "losing credibility" or being revealed as a fraud, their ability to affect positive change in their clients is enhanced. There is an authentic, extremely compassionate (often humorous) feel to an ACT session when the therapist is holding to the model. It is a relief that we can all just be human. It is also a revelation about just how powerful being a human can be when we stop trying not to have what we have, and instead work on how we want to show up in the world.

ACT Enhances Individual Learning

When several individuals come together to learn something, more learning opportunities are created for everyone. Members learn from one another both in terms of mutual feedback and also from being privy to their peers' learning process. In ACT this is particularly the case because the core processes targeted in sessions are common to all. Each member will be somewhere along the continuum of psychological flexibility at any point in time. So it is not necessary that members relate to the content of a peer's words or struggles. The processes in play will apply to each member's personal struggle regardless, and indeed to what each is experiencing at any point in the group session. In short, what is being worked on is directly applicable to everyone at all times. And because these core processes are ubiquitous, there will be many, many examples of how they show up in our lives. That's a pretty big learning opportunity!

While a group setting provides fertile ground for developing all the core processes in ACT, we will highlight defusion as one that is particularly aided by the group work. That is, helping some clients defuse from thoughts can be a real challenge. When someone is particularly fused with what his mind is handing him, it is difficult to help him see that he is fused. Some defusing is required to recognize fusion as it occurs. This may be why our clients often learn best from third person examples when they are really stuck on something. Even if highly fused herself, a group member can recognize how fusion is showing up for a peer with the therapist's help. Once she understands what is actually meant by "being fused with thoughts" and sees how that manifests in others, she is better able to apply that process to herself.

There is another level of learning available in group therapy. We can also take the group itself as an entity that is progressing (or devolving) along the continuum of psychological flexibility. Is the group as a whole heading into stuff (defusion, willingness, values action)? Has the group spent most of the session problem solving and trying to figure out why a member is angry with his wife (fusion, unwillingness, self-as-content)? Is there a stilted, unsatisfying feel to the session because of something unsaid (avoidance/unwillingness)? The bottom line is that on top of the many clinical opportunities happening at the individual level, the therapist can point to and work with the processes as they apply to the group as a whole. This is why we love doing ACT in groups. Opportunities abound!

ACT Harnesses Social Support

Much has been written about the benefits of social support, so we'll not revisit that here. Rather, we point to ways in which ACT optimizes the support available in a group therapy setting. For one, members learn to be better present to their peers, creating an opening for empathy. An important thrust of the therapy is that we are working on what it means to be human, as opposed to trying to solve problems or rectify certain diagnoses, symptoms, and the like. As we've discussed at length, the core processes of ACT are common to all, and participants easily connect over the shared struggle of being human.

Along with learning to be present in groups, members also learn to be willing to experience what is there to be had. When combined with the commonality of the struggle, being willing enables participants to experience discomfort and, thus, each other's pain. The abilities targeted in ACT also foster group participation. Members learn to defuse from what their minds are telling them about speaking up (*This will sound stupid; I need to know exactly what to say*).

Finally, there is evidence now that our ability to reach personal goals is increased when we have people in our lives who support our efforts (Dailey, Crook, Glowacki, Prenger, & Winslow, 2016). The success of Alcoholics Anonymous and similar groups is a good example of how this can work in a group setting. In ACT, clients are guided to identify their values in various life domains as well as specific goals that take them in these valued directions. Especially when the therapist helps articulate the shared values of the group—the intention to learn how to better their lives, for example—group members learn to see such moves as examples of valued action. As all members join in the effort to "live according to their values," they support each other and themselves in living life vitally and well.

ACT Facilitates Compassion

In our discussion of social support we mentioned that ACT can engender empathy. Difficulties are phrased as *human* difficulties, and learning to be present to that struggle helps group members contact a sense of compassion for their shared experience. ACT also has important implications when it comes to self-compassion. We have found it interesting, and sobering, that so many individuals demonstrate or report an inability to have compassion for themselves. In fact, many clients state that while they have compassion for others, they are absolutely unable to find compassion for themselves.

The fundamental principles in ACT can be of great assistance with this issue. For one thing, it would be inconsistent with the model (not to mention futile) to suggest that clients need to be able to somehow manufacture the feeling of self-compassion. Similarly, providing "evidence" for their deservedness—all the reasons they are worthy of compassion—also contradicts the model. In ACT we seek to alter the function rather than the form of thoughts and feelings. These clients have established a relational network around "self-compassion" that is here to stay. However, we can help such clients notice what their minds hand them around self-compassion and learn to hold that more lightly. And there is this: when we stop striving for the emotional experience of compassion and instead learn radical self-acceptance (accepting ourselves fully, which in this case would include the experience of not feeling compassionate toward oneself), the feeling of self-compassion might in fact show up.

Here is another key distinction: In ACT we view emotions as part of an unfolding stream of experiences. We do not hold the idea that certain ones are good and others are bad, or that we can arrive at the desirable ones as we can a destination (e.g., achieving happiness). Rather, feelings come and go, adding richness, depth, vitality, and yes, pain, to our lives. So in ACT we aim not so much for the feeling of self-compassion, but rather for self-compassion as a stance, or an action. We might ask our client, "If you were *being* compassionate toward yourself, what might that look like?" Treating oneself kindly, even if the internal experience is one of judgment or unworthiness, *is* within the client's grasp.

As it applies to group work, *being* compassionate might include refraining from issuing harsh judgments (verbally, that is, as judgmental thoughts and feelings could well show up) and actively listening to one's peers. As it pertains to self, it might involve noticing and defusing from self-judgments and making room for what one is experiencing.

ACT Assists *with* Problematic Responses

Just as groups can be powerful vehicles for positive change, they can be powerful vehicles for staying stuck. Members can behave in ways that stifle growth for the entire group and can facilitate behaviors that run counter to what they are hoping to accomplish. Even the best intentions can result in dynamics that are problematic, and looking through that ACT lens helps therapists recognize when "helping" is actually standing in the way. In fact, the model not only illuminates problematic group dynamics, but also offers a way to work with these in ways that increase group members' psychological flexibility. We have devoted chapter 3 to exploring this important feature of ACT in more detail.

ACT Fosters *Constructive Feedback*

Let's look again at the learning mechanisms available in groups. One of the greatest offerings of a group setting is interpersonal feedback. In chapter 1 we examined how languaging can cause us to dwell in a verbal virtual reality, and that a cost is awareness of what is occurring in our actual lives. If we were actively tracking how our behavior was functioning, for example, we might notice that we weren't really listening to someone and that authentic connection was therefore lacking. Or perhaps we might notice that although feeling vulnerable seems intolerable, we are, in fact, able to hold that experience. The therapy group provides a context wherein it is permissible, even desirable, for members to articulate how they experience each other. This provides invaluable information to participants; essentially, members track for one another how their behavior functions in the group. The group setting also provides ample opportunities for natural consequences of behavior to occur in that workable behavior is socially reinforced and unworkable behavior is socially ineffective.

The core processes in ACT serve to enhance this potential learning mechanism. For example, in learning to defuse from thoughts, members gain important space between what their minds are telling them and how they then respond. The therapist facilitates and models being present, willingness, defusion, self-as-context, values, and committed action—all of which serve to make interpersonal feedback fruitful. For example, rather than making a comment such as "You don't respect what others have to say," a member might learn to offer, "When you said that just then I had the thought that you don't respect me. I felt really frustrated." Notice that not only does the member being referred to receive important feedback, but all the core processes are nicely modeled for the group.

Summary

In this chapter we have explored some of the gifts ACT brings to the table in therapy that are magnified in a group setting. If we have implied that ACT is the only therapy that offers benefits to groups, however, we have erred. Our position is that ACT is particularly good at harnessing the mechanisms of therapeutic change. In illuminating and targeting the processes that uniquely define the human experience—both our suffering and our incredible capabilities—we set ourselves up to maximize the opportunity that exists when people come together with the intention to grow.

CHAPTER 3

Using ACT to Turn Challenges into Opportunity

If you are familiar with group work, you are well acquainted with the most obvious source of difficulty: a lot is going on! Each group member brings his history to the group, each will react and respond accordingly, and each will influence the others in the group and the therapy as it unfolds. And of course as the number of participants grows, complexity increases and the session pace can start jumping. With all this, there is greater potential for problematic dynamics to develop. The good news? The complexity of group therapy is where the ACT model can really assist therapists. It's as though there's all this stuff flying around the room, but when you look a little closer, you see it is all connected to six basic strands that can be gathered up and used to make sense of things. Regardless of what shows up in the room, the core processes will apply. In this chapter we will demonstrate how working at the process level helps the therapist sift through everything that's going on and intervene effectively.

A related point is that looking at what occurs in group through an ACT lens helps turn therapeutic challenges into therapeutic fodder. Even a very perplexing response or disruptive behavior can be used to further the processes targeted in ACT. This makes sense when we remember that ability with the processes is on a continuum and can manifest as a strength or a deficit to varying degrees. Simply helping the group recognize a deficit in one instance (e.g., engaging in avoidance strategies rather than choosing to be willing) can facilitate growth in that very area.

There's no doubt there is a learning curve to becoming competent in ACT. Once therapists have developed some capacity with it, however, they often report feeling more "free" in their therapy sessions. One reason for this is that working within the model takes therapists out of the bind they can find themselves in with other modalities. For example, we have discussed that one of the challenges ACT therapists face is learning to let discomfort be rather than trying to fix whatever's going on. That also can be quite freeing. When we consider the futility of trying to help group members have different thoughts, feelings, and sensations (the very agenda that has likely been keeping them stuck), it is no small thing to recognize that fixing is not what is needed.

Another reason conducting ACT can be freeing is that the model directly applies to the therapist as well. We recognize that just as trying to fix the internal experiences of group members is both futile and unnecessary, so too is trying to fix whatever the therapist is experiencing. All is welcome at the table. That means the ACT therapist can have her frustration, dislike, boredom—all those experiences we are quick to judge as being "nontherapeutic." Such experiences are a part of interacting with other human beings and do not need to be gone in order to engage effectively. We can *be* compassionate, fair, and respectful regardless of the thoughts and feelings going on. By bringing acceptance to our own experience, we are freed up to engage in the session according to our values.

In this chapter we'll talk about how some of the principal difficulties that come with conducting any therapy in a group setting can be addressed from within an ACT framework. Some issues are more about the therapist; some manifest at an individual level; some can be viewed as group-level difficulties. (This categorization method is purely for practical purposes, as anything that happens in the group is part of a larger context. An issue that involves a particular group member, for example, is the result of any number of contextual variables and influences the larger group context in turn.) We know we can only skim the surface of all the ways group dynamics can be challenging, but we hope this discussion will help demonstrate how ACT lends itself well to working through them.

Therapist Challenges

In this section we will address some of the ways in which therapists can stand in the way of the therapy. We anticipate that as we move through these difficulties you will notice commonalities. You will see how one misstep can lead to another, for example, or how avoidance might be at work in several of these therapist-related challenges. If we do our job, you will also begin to notice that despite the innumerable ways these difficulties can manifest, you can turn to the core ACT processes for guidance.

Content Versus Process

We touch again upon the importance of working at a process rather than content level (or of working with *function* rather than *form*). This is arguably the most fundamental clinical guideline, and one of the hardest to master. It is astoundingly easy to get hooked into content. Fastening on content is what our minds are geared to do. However, it is safe to say that if a therapist is stuck, it is likely because he is stymied by trying to address content—to problem solve, to fix what can't be fixed—or is just being pulled off track. Shifting to process (or function) can get things moving again.

Barry: So what's next?

Therapist: Next?

Barry: So what do we do? Where are we going with this?

Therapist: You mean with this therapy?

Barry: Yeah. I understand what you're saying about looking *at* thoughts and not just *from* thoughts—I think. So…now what?

Therapist: So now we can see thoughts as thoughts, as something that's going on.

Barry: Okaaaay… So what do I do with that? I'm not sure what this is supposed to do.

And it continues. Now let's work at the process level:

Barry: So what's next?

Therapist: Next?

Barry: So what do we do? Where are we going with this?

Therapist: You mean with this therapy?

Barry: Yeah. I understand what you're saying about looking *at* thoughts and not just *from* thoughts—I think. So…now what?

Therapist: (*pausing to contact the present, slowing things down*) Hmmm. Can I just ask what you are experiencing right now?

Barry: Right now?

Therapist: Yeah, what's going on for you in this moment?

Barry: I dunno…I feel antsy…I'm not sure where we're headed with all this.

Therapist: Yeah (*unhurried*). So antsy…sort of on edge or anxious?

               (*Barry nods.*)

Therapist: And can I ask you whether this is something you do when you're feeling antsy or anxious?

Barry: What do you mean?

Therapist:	You are feeling on edge, antsy…and so you are asking questions, trying to figure things out.
Barry:	(*thinks*) Yeah, I guess…I don't like it. Oh, so I'm trying to control.
Therapist:	(*to group*) Let's just notice how that works. This is a great example of what we do, isn't it? We feel antsy or anxious or uncomfortable in some way and our minds get busy trying to fix it somehow. (*pausing to let the moment settle*) So maybe we can use this as an opportunity to do something else! Let's take a few moments to notice what is going on for us in this moment (*pause*). Let's see if we can notice and gently hold whatever it is that we're experiencing. (*Therapist then falls silent and models just sitting and noticing for a minute or two.*)

Though certainly pulled to address Barry's concerns at a content level, the therapist stays on course and creates an opportunity to further the work.

Teaching/Telling Versus Doing

Another common therapist misstep is approaching ACT didactically at the cost of experiential learning. It is extremely easy for therapists to fall into a mode where they are "telling the therapy" rather than bringing it to life in the room. Let's look at some contributing factors:

FUSION WITH RULES

One of the reasons therapists can overtalk in session is that they are fused with rules rather than attending to what is actually unfolding. For example, the therapist might believe it is necessary to cover the material as planned for the session, or that the group "must" understand and buy in to a particular idea. It's not that rules are bad, by the way, but that being rigidly attached to them can be costly. If we are caught up in rules about what *needs* to happen in the session, we are less aware of what is *actually* happening. In the pursuit of ideas, we miss in-the-moment opportunities to work with the core processes present in the session.

We see here the importance of therapists being able to employ the very processes they are hoping to impart to the group. We can't erase the rules in our heads, we can't stop our minds from coming up with them, but we can see them for what they are. This requires contacting the present with willingness to have what is there, and being able to notice and defuse from the thoughts (including rules) going on. We can now expand that present-moment awareness to function. In this case, we can assess how our overtalking is actually functioning in the room. Because we have defused from the rules, they have less influence over our behavior and we can make the choice to do something else (i.e., we can contact the present, choose to be willing, experience self-as-context, and choose a committed action that is in line with our values).

ENTHUSIASM

Overteaching/telling in ACT can also arise from simple enthusiasm. The therapist is excited about ACT and what it offers, and very much wants the group to "get it" and start reaping benefits. Rather than allowing the therapeutic process to unfold, the therapist verbally dumps "The Story of ACT" in members' laps—and then wonders why it doesn't result in behavior change. We recognize that it is quite satisfying to have answers and to "help" people, though in ACT this very desire can work against the therapy. Therapists can easily fall into persuading or convincing, which then teeters into a right/wrong dynamic that counteracts psychological flexibility.

Contacting one's own experience and choosing to be willing is again helpful here. Enthusiasm and eagerness can bring vitality to the work if it doesn't lead the therapist to force the therapy. The task is to notice and hold this desire to just tell ACT to the group, to notice and hold the urges and impatience enthusiasm can bring. The therapist can notice her eagerness and yet choose to just rest in the moment. Remembering that notions of right and wrong are language based and taught, she can hold more lightly her own notions that ACT is the "right" way to go. This enables her to be more present to the group and where members are in the therapy, and to then intervene in a way that will help them move forward.

Therapist:	(*stopping herself suddenly*) You know, I just want to stop for a moment and notice what's happening in this moment (*pauses and takes a few unhurried breaths as group members wait*). Can I ask what's happening for you all? What are you experiencing?
	(*Group members look at one another.*)
Therapist:	I just realized I was doing a lot of talking. Like I'm trying to convince you of something. (*pauses again as she allows herself to get present*) I notice some anxiety…some worries about how this is going over, all that sort of stuff… Can I ask what is going on for you?
Gina:	I feel sort of confused.
Gary:	I get what you're saying, but I don't know…I'm just not very into this today. (*Other group members nod.*)
Therapist:	Yes. There definitely seems to be that stuff in the room. And did you notice what I did? I got really busy trying to fix it or ignore it or something. And it was there anyway! (*Group laughs.*)

Therapist: Let's shift gears and do a mindfulness exercise. Let's just get present to what's here, but in a noticing rather than fixing way. And notice, too, how we can choose to engage even though we've got thoughts and feelings going on about not being into it and so on.

Rigid Attachment to the Expert Role

Now we turn to the issue of therapists being overly attached to their role as mental health experts. This can happen in part for reasons we have already mentioned, such as being fused with rules or avoiding discomfort. Not only is hanging on to the expert role a common misstep in ACT, but its effects can be insidious, subtly (or not so subtly) working against the therapy.

In chapter 8 we will explore self-as-context and how we apply ACT to help group members develop more flexible ways of experiencing themselves. In short, we aim to help them contact the self that is larger than their constructed identities, that is more than all the categorizations and evaluations they learned to apply to themselves. This frees them from needing to defend or disprove their self-concepts, and helps them see that their choices in life need not be constrained by their self-perceptions. Therapists, too, are less constrained when they understand that the various roles they assume are verbal constructions—workable in some instances, less so in others. One of the drawbacks in assuming an expert role when doing ACT is that it can strengthen problematic associations group members may have about themselves and being in therapy. For example, group members may self-identify as patients, as being sick, as needing to be fixed by someone who is not similarly broken. These self-conceptions run counter to the tenets of ACT. Even the most well-intentioned therapist can inadvertently support these perceptions by operating within the Expert role.

Additionally, there is an inherent contradiction in the expert/patient dynamic when it comes to this model. ACT assumes a level playing field between therapists and group members (derived from fundamental principles of behavior that apply to us all). So, while the therapist does have something to offer the group—familiarity with a technology that group members may find helpful—he faces the same struggles of being human. He may have expertise in ACT, but Expert as an identity is neither needed nor helpful.

Being Right/Persuading

It is easy to fall prey to the necessity of being right if one is attached to being the Expert. Even if the intention is to help the group, the implied message is that the therapist knows best, that group members are wrong and misguided, and that there are right ways of being and the group isn't there. When fused with the notion of self as expert, therapists are more prone to push their own agendas onto the group, when what we are after in ACT is helping group members identify and pursue their own values in life. Then there's the fact that debating, convincing, and persuading just don't seem to work too well.

If we remember the trickiness of language, we can see such notions of right/wrong as being learned rather than "truth." We are guided to offer ACT as an approach to living that we believe the group will find helpful, not as a "should." We can notice our desire to be right and all-knowing (and our thoughts about what it means if we are *not*) while doing what works.

Dan:	(*arms crossed, looking and sounding a little hostile*) You said that using control strategies doesn't work, but mine work lots of times.
Therapist:	How do they work?
Dan:	I control my anger all the time. Believe me, you wouldn't want me to stop doing that!
Therapist:	But does your anger really go away when you do that?
Dan:	It stays under control.
Therapist:	But it's still there.
Dan:	(*voice rising a little*) Are you saying I should stop controlling it? Just lash out and do whatever?
Therapist:	There's a difference between what you're feeling on the inside and what you do.
Dan:	And what I'm *doing* is controlling my anger.
Therapist:	(*stopping herself suddenly and pausing for a moment*) I'm pausing because I'm noticing what's happening here. (*pauses again as she contacts her experience, continues unhurriedly*) I feel sort of tense, and…a sense of pressure. I'm noticing a need to be right about this… (*to group*) Did you sense that as well? (*Group members nod.*) Yeah (*to Dan*), there's this need going on to convince you or something. [*The therapist is modeling contacting the present, willingness to have what's there to be had and to be vulnerable, and self-as-process. She elicits participation from the larger group to augment this modeling and to shift out of the one-on-one struggle with Dan.*]
	(*Dan looks a bit off-guard, is silent.*)
Therapist:	Did anyone else notice what you were feeling as Dan and I were talking? What was going on for you? [*The therapist uses this opportunity to help group members build self-as-process and defusion. She is also turning to the group in the hopes that their modeling of the processes will help Dan get unstuck.*]

Gina:	I got anxious! (*A couple other members nod.*)
Mary:	I wanted the group to be over—in fact I checked the clock to see how much time was left!
Gary:	I was getting really impatient, like "Let's just move on!"
Therapist:	How great that you were able to catch all that! Isn't it something, though? All that stuff pops up instantaneously. And there's also a sense of how easily Dan and I could have just kept on going, right? (*Group members nod.*) We could still be at it, which probably wouldn't do much for anyone here.

In this example the therapist drew upon all the core ACT processes. She contacted the present from a stance of willingness, noticed the various thoughts, feelings, and sensations going on for her (self-as-process, self-as-context), openly claimed them (willingness, defusion, values, committed action) and used them to further the therapy. In essence, she used what was happening in the room to demonstrate the very ideas she had been hoping to impart to Gary at a more content level: that we can simply notice our internal experiences and choose to engage in workable behaviors despite the presence of difficult thoughts and feelings.

Avoidance

In our years of supervising and training others in ACT, we find avoidance at the heart of many clinical missteps. For example, we have mentioned overtalking as problematic; often therapists resort to talking as a response to something uncomfortable going on in the room, some emotional upset, maybe just silence. We have observed many therapists start talking *more* as they sense a disconnect with what they're saying, as though they can somehow verbally force things to come around. Telling jokes, changing the subject, ignoring a subject—there are numerous ways therapist avoidance can show up in a session.

When it comes to being entrenched in the role of Expert, avoidance is often a key culprit. Specifically, therapists are working to mitigate the discomfort of uncertainty, of confusion, of being personally vulnerable, of being "found out" as a fraud. This discomfort can be particularly strong if therapists have been trained in models that advise against self-disclosure in therapy or other forms of "crossing boundaries." Interacting in a more equal, human-to-human way with group members can feel very strange and even unsafe.

With this comes another opportunity to walk the walk in ACT, and to use one's own experience in the room as a means to further the therapy. There is no need for any of this to be gone. Our desire to be comfortable, to be wise, to be impervious or immune can be in the room. The key is to claim it, accept it, and then do what works (i.e., contact the present, choose to be willing, defuse from unworkable rules, notice the self-as-context, and engage in the group according to your values as an ACT therapist).

No Oomph

One of the more miserable experiences for group therapists is a flat session. Most of us have been there at one point or another, where things just aren't flowing, nothing's happening, and group members are not engaged (we can say bored). Let's look at a few reasons this can occur from an ACT perspective:

WORKING TOO HARD

This is related to talking/telling the therapy, being right, and being fused with rules. If the therapist is working harder than anyone else in the group, she may be trying to fix or compensate for what is occurring in the moment (e.g., nonengagement by the group). She may be focused on content to the point where the session has become "heady," squeezing out awareness of experience and the vitality that brings. If therapists get the sense they are working very hard, that is a cue to stop, contact the present, and make room for what has shown up.

NOT BEING AUTHENTIC

We can again point to holding on to the expert role, fusion with rules, and avoidance as barriers to therapists engaging with their group in an authentic manner. There are few things more alive than genuine, human connection—yet it can be so elusive! Many therapists fear being seen in all their fallibility, as though their perceived flaws will decrease their credibility and worth as therapists. However, it is that very shared humanity that helps group members come forward, to see themselves in others and open up to learning. It is in authentic connection that we learn genuine acceptance of ourselves and of others. Finally, being inauthentic doesn't tend to work, in that at some level the group knows what's going on. The therapist may be striving to be perceived in a certain way, but what the group is attuned to is the striving itself.

STAYING WITH CONTENT OVER PROCESS

We have discussed the importance of working with the core processes and won't revisit that here. We simply point out that content is by its very verbal nature "in the head," whereas process, or experiential learning, is alive and in the room. It is possible to fall into a mode where the therapy becomes a lifeless exchange of information rather than about doing and experiencing. One of the easiest ways to bring life to a session is to move to process. This can be done in a number of ways, but one of the most rapid methods is to drop to one's own experience in the room.

Imagine a scenario where the therapist has been talking away for much of the session and has not managed to get any real participation from the group:

Therapist: (*stopping suddenly and looking around the room*) Wow, am I bored!

              (*Group members, shocked, are suddenly all attentive.*)

Therapist: I've been talking away in here, but it feels like nothing much is happening. Does it feel like that to you? (*A few members nod hesitantly.*)

Therapist: Yeah. And the more I've sensed that, the harder I've tried to talk it away. But I imagine that gets *really* boring! (*looks inquisitively at the group, more members nod*)

Therapist: (*curiously*) So what do you all do with it? (*Members look confused.*) What have you been experiencing as I've just rambled on today?

Dan: I don't know. I'm just not getting it or something.

Mary: I can't really concentrate. I didn't sleep well last night. (*Other members nod.*)

Therapist: And did you notice what you did with that? So confusion or not getting it shows up, being tired and difficulty with concentrating…how did you respond to that stuff when it showed up in here?

Mary: I sort of tuned out.

Gary: I just didn't want to be here today.

Therapist: Oh, kind of like, I'm not into it so I'll tune out, just sit back. (*Several group members nod.*)

Therapist: And notice how we all sort of coped with what was happening in here in our own ways, but the result wasn't very satisfying. At least it wasn't for me! (*Group members nod again, clearly more attentive and engaged at this point.*)

Therapist: I'd like to invite us all to do something here. Something different. Let's start by acknowledging to ourselves what we're feeling and thinking in here; let's make room for it (*pauses to allow the group time to do this*). And then let's choose to engage in spite of it all. That is, in the few minutes we have left, let's be here fully—with our fatigue, with our confusion, even our boredom. We can have all that going on, and still choose to engage with each other in this moment in time. Are you with me? (*Members agree.*) I'll wrap up with a mindfulness exercise so we can put this into practice.

PLAYING IT SAFE

As you may have guessed, avoidance is at the heart of this misstep. Playing it safe can take the form of following a script in session as a crutch to avoid the discomfort of not knowing what to do or of stumbling in session. It can mean not speaking to what's in the room because it's uncomfortable. It can mean using the same tired exercises and metaphors rather than trying something new. These are just some of the ways therapists can play it safe and miss out on the full potential of this therapy. Attachment to the expert role, fusion with rules about what it means to be competent (and to fail)— these can cause therapists to hang on to what they know rather than being open to new opportunities. When we understand that being the assured, smooth, competent therapist is more our deal (i.e., our attachment to a conceptualized self), we can choose to make moves that are more about what might benefit the group. We can try that new exercise and see what happens next.

Group Member Challenges

In this section, we turn to difficulties individual group members can raise in a group setting. Although we will touch on only a few examples here, we will show how the same six ACT processes offer useful conceptualizations of what is happening in the room and, more importantly, suggest ways to effectively intervene.

Story Telling

It is not uncommon to have a group member who frequently derails the work by interjecting personal stories. Function is our guide here. That is, there is nothing inherently bad about telling stories! However, if it obstructs meaningful work, pushes people away, or prevents being in the moment, it can be problematic. Looking through that ACT lens, we can hypothesize that a group member who engages in excessive story telling might have deficits in contacting the present and/or being willing to have what's there to be had in the present. He might be so fused with his thoughts that he isn't tracking the consequences of his behavior (e.g., that he has taken the group off course, that his peers are bored or frustrated). He may be rigidly attached to a conceptualized self and all the stories about that self (e.g., as a war veteran). It may be that the individual desires connection and resorts to this sort of sharing as a way to connect. Regardless, learning to contact the present, to defuse from thoughts, and experience self-as-process and self-as-context would help this individual detach from his stories and better track his behavior and its effects upon the group.

Therapist:	(*interrupting Barry as he's telling a story*) Barry, do you mind if I interrupt you for a moment?
Barry:	Uh, no.
Therapist:	What are you experiencing right now? (*The therapist is helping Barry to defuse from his thoughts about the past and contact the present.*)
Barry:	Um…I don't know…
Therapist:	Can you say why you are wanting to tell the group this story? What is it that you are wanting the group to know? (*This pulls for contacting the present, self-as-process, and considering function.*)
Barry:	I'm not really sure…
Therapist:	Well, let's just pause a moment and see if we can notice what's happening (*pauses, takes a few deep breathes*). What are you feeling? (*contacting the present, willingness, defusing, self-as-context, and self-as-process*)
Barry:	I feel sort of anxious now.
Therapist:	Yeah, like if you get out of the story and get *here*, anxiety shows up. (*self-as-process*)
Barry:	Yeah. I'm not even sure why I was telling that story now…
Therapist:	(*to group*) I wonder if you all could share what you were experiencing when Barry was talking. *The therapist is using group feedback to help Barry track how his behavior functions in the group.*
Dan:	(*after a pause*) To be honest, I was irritated. I mean, I like Barry and everything, but he's always going off on his stories and it gets kinda old.
Therapist:	Thanks for taking a risk and sharing that Dan, but I'd like for you guys to speak directly to Barry.
Mary:	(*to Barry*) I'd rather just hear more about *you*. I know all these stories but it seems like I don't know *you*.

And so on. Therapist style is critical here. That is, by tone and manner, the therapist conveys compassion and a genuine desire for understanding Barry. While straightforward about what is happening in the room, the therapist is careful to convey that the point is to learn and help one another grow.

Being a Victim

We refer to the individual who steadfastly perceives himself as being wronged as being powerless. This particular presentation suggests rigid attachment to a conceptualized self (e.g., as "Victim"), which in turn suggests useful work might be done with self-as-process and self-as-context (both of which loosen up self-as-*content*). Examining the function of holding this perspective will be important. For example, being helpless may function as a way to avoid personal responsibility and risk of failure. If so, it would be useful to develop willingness and the ability to defuse from thoughts. Such an individual could benefit from connecting with personal values that would encourage more agency in his life.

Therapist:	Gina, what happened just now? You were talking and then it seems like you shut down. (*self as process, contacting the present, pointing to function.*)
Gina:	(*reluctantly*) There's obviously no point.
Therapist:	No point?
Gina:	Everything I say in here gets turned around. Nobody cares what I have to say anyway.
Therapist:	Those are really painful thoughts! What sorts of feelings show up when you have thoughts like that? (*defusion, self as process*)
Gina:	I don't feel anything. Besides, what's the point?
Therapist:	So at times like that you feel nothing, and then you have that thought again: What's the point? (*Gina nods again.*) [*Rather than get caught up in the content of Gina's response, "I don't feel anything," the therapist sticks with self-as-process and places "feeling nothing" as part of the ongoing experience.*]
Therapist:	Yeah, no fun! And how does that stop you? Do you buy the thought that there's no point? (*self as process, defusion*)
Gina:	There is no point!

Therapist:	(*nodding understandingly*) Got it. There it is again—no point. And I want to acknowledge you for what you're doing right now. (*defusion*)
Gina:	What do you mean?
Therapist:	You've shared some of what you deal with at times like this. Really painful, hopeless thoughts and feelings. And it sounds like at times like this you buy what your mind hands you and just want to give up. And yet, in this moment you are not allowing that to stop you. You have been hanging in there with me and engaging anyway, even though your mind is telling you there's no point. That's pretty cool. (*self-as-process, defusion, self as context*, and *good old-fashioned positive reinforcement*)

No Trust

It is not uncommon for group members to report having difficulty trusting others. This is often laid out as a barrier to group participation, and it frequently contains an explicit or implied challenge to the other group members—that they and the therapist need to somehow prove they are trustworthy.

Again, the principles of ACT are helpful here. We can see how fusion and rigid rule following are at work here and can help the group (and ourselves) defuse from unhelpful notions about trust. Trust as a thing to somehow acquire and keep (or lose) is not attainable even if we *were* somehow able to pass a trust test. Trust is a construct and does not physically exist. We experience feelings of trust and distrust that come and go. Trust as an action, however, is a choice we can make. Taking a risk and sharing something despite not knowing what the future holds (e.g., how others will respond) is an example of *being* trusting and does not actually require the *feeling* of trust.

So the ACT therapist would not need to work at the content level here. Rather than engage in what is sure to be unproductive problem solving around the member's feelings of distrust, we would look to see how this behavior—sharing that he does not trust the other group members—is functioning in the moment. For example, is he avoiding? Does setting up this sort of barrier serve to keep discomfort away or does it let him off the hook for fully participating in therapy? Is he thinking that his feelings of distrust need to be eliminated or at least lessened before he will be "okay" in the group?

Depending on our hypotheses as to how this is currently functioning, we are then guided as to what might productively move things forward. For example, we could use this opportunity to foster defusion (noticing the distrust), or being willing despite feeling distrustful, or perhaps taking valued action. That is, despite the thoughts and feelings of distrust going on, what choice might the client make that takes him closer to, rather than further from, his values?

Jr. Therapist

Sometimes group members take on the role of Jr. Therapist, "helping" the therapist rather than simply participating as another member of the group. This can be particularly problematic when the individual thinks she has a grasp on things but does not. If we consider function, it could be that the individual gains a sense of satisfaction from being in a position of knowing. A deficit in being present and self-as-process could be preventing her from tracking how her behavior is actually affecting the group. It could be that she has established an identity around being the person with the answers, or the person who can help. This would suggest attachment to a conceptualized self, and fusion with rules. It could be that she is feeling a lot of excitement about the work and wants her peers to benefit from the therapy. Helping her contact the present and explore what she is experiencing (self-as-process) will help illuminate the function of her behavior. It would then be useful to explore whether or not her behavior is actually working, and what she might do that is more in line with her desire to be helpful in the group.

Rescuer/Caretaker

Many individuals have self-concepts (e.g., as caretaker, as "nice") that create rigid rules around what is and is not acceptable behavior. For example, a nice group member might have difficulty offering anything but positive feedback. It is often uncomfortable to witness another's discomfort, and group members will often engage in "rescuing" in an attempt to mitigate their own experience. In terms of the core processes, this points to attachment with a conceptualized self, fusion with rules, difficulties with contacting the present, and deficits in willingness.

Although particular individuals may be prone to be caretaking of other members, this is a common phenomenon in groups as a whole. We address this further in the "Collusion" section below and provide a working example there.

Group Level Challenges

In the previous sections we talked about some of the things therapists and individual group members can do that stand in the way of the therapy. In this section we will take a step back and consider group functioning at a meta-level.

We can often accomplish more by intervening at a group level. For one thing, we harness the social factors that shape behavior. Even a very stuck group member can start to move when the larger group shows the way. When we point to things at a group level, we can circumvent some of the barriers that can arise when we work with individuals. While feedback is no less pertinent, it can feel less personal and members can be more open to learning when approached in this way.

Avoidance

Just as we seek to help group members recognize avoidance and its potential costs when it arises, it is useful to point out when the group as a whole is avoiding. (We assure you that if you are looking you will find it frequently!)

Therapist:	Did you all notice what just happened? (*Group members are curious, unsure.*) We started to touch something a little painful, and then immediately moved off the topic.
Or:	
Therapist:	I just realized we are all problem solving right now, trying to "help" Gary rather than just allowing him to have his feelings around this.

There are certain points in the therapy where avoidance at a group level is likely to show up. We certainly see this early on, when group members have yet to learn the abilities that will help them choose willingness in the place of avoidance. Simply the prospect of contacting the moment (and all its grief, sorrow, fear, regret, and self-loathing) can be terrifying. So we do anticipate that the group as a whole will be initially avoidant, and we work with this by gradually helping members contact the present and learn to hold what is there.

Another point where avoidance can show up is less intuitive. It often appears as the group has developed some ability to defuse from thoughts and is starting to grasp self-as-context. There is a realization among members that if they aren't their thoughts and feelings, if thoughts and feelings aren't in charge, they can no longer be used as excuses for not living. Yikes. There is often profound grief as members realize they have lost years to fighting an unnecessary battle.

Navigating this can be tricky. It is important that the therapist demonstrate compassion for the bind the group is in while also helping members hold their fears or grief in a workable way. That is, they *are* responsible for the choices they make in life, *and* the fear and worry that can come with this are natural and don't need to be fixed. Their minds might hand them thoughts about wasted years. Nonetheless, the question before them remains: what will you do from this moment forward?

Passivity

Earlier we pointed out how therapists can contribute to group passivity by approaches such as teaching/telling the therapy. However, group members can bring this element to the therapy all on their own, and it can be a tough nut to crack. Besides all of the good reasons there could be to avoid participating, engaging is simply effortful. Why not sit back and just observe?

One way we work with this is to behave as though we fully expect participation from the group. We will ask a question, for example, and then wait expectantly. We will sit for as long as it takes. Trust us, eventually someone will become so uncomfortable with the silence she will speak up. We then move on but do the same thing throughout the session as needed (ask a question and wait for participation). This essentially shapes the group's behavior—nonparticipation is linked with being uncomfortable (or alternatively, nonparticipation doesn't "work" as desired). This requires willingness on the part of the therapist—it's uncomfortable for him too. But the message it sends is clear, that being in the group is about *being* in the group.

Another way to work with group passivity is to address it directly:

| Therapist: | I notice that no one is responding to my questions; no one is really participating today. It feels sort of strange in here—as though there's something unsaid. (*looks expectantly at the group*) Is there something in here that needs to be said? (*waits*) |

Or

| Therapist: | I feel very stuck. I'm not sure where to go. (*Group is silent.*) I could keep trying to fix it, but I suspect that would result in more of the same. (*Group waits.*) So I think that my task is to just be here and notice what it's like to be stuck. (*sits silently*) |

Finally, the experiential exercises in ACT can be useful here. By their very nature, they elicit active participation, and experiential learning can occur regardless of the thoughts and feelings going on. We often use nonparticipation as a cue that an experiential exercise is in order.

Collusion

Group members can support each other, console each other, lift each other up, and spur each other on. They can also collude in behaviors that keep each other stuck. We can see this sort of enabling throughout the therapy, particularly when group members are struggling. There can be a sense that "support" means aligning with each other, even if that entails supporting the very behaviors that have proved problematic. It is helpful to tag this the moment it appears.

Therapist:	Okay, let's review the values sheets I handed out last week. Dan, would you like to go first? What was it like for you to work on that?
Dan:	(*looking uncomfortable*) Oh, I didn't do it.
Therapist:	Ah. What was that about?

Dan:	I don't know…I thought about it…
Therapist:	So you were thinking about it…then what happened?
Dan:	(*a little tense*) I don't know! I just forgot!
Mary:	I forgot too!
Gina:	Me too.
Gary:	I have enough going on, it's hard enough to make time to come in here. I don't have time for paperwork stuff too.
Therapist:	Looks like this values task brought up a lot of stuff! (*Group is silent.*) From forgetting, to thoughts about not having time… Mary, can I ask what was going on for you a moment ago? What were you experiencing when I was asking Dan about the values sheet?
Mary:	I felt bad for him!
Therapist:	I see. You were feeling bad for him…as though he was in trouble?
Mary:	Yes. I could see he felt bad about not doing the homework, but you kept asking him about it.
Therapist:	Is that why you jumped in to say you had forgotten as well?
Mary:	I wanted him to know he wasn't alone—wanted *you* to know he wasn't alone.
Therapist:	I see, you wanted to help him. (*to the rest of the group*) Was that going on for you as well? (*Group nods.*) Is it safe to say you were also helping yourselves? That is, it was hard for you to experience what you were experiencing when I was talking with Dan, so you wanted to stop the conversation? (*Members think it over, nod.*)
Therapist:	(*to group*) I want to acknowledge your caring for Dan, and also how hard it is to feel this stuff sometimes. (*pause*) At the same time, I'd like you to stop for a moment and consider what you actually think about that task. That is, do you think completing that worksheet might have offered something to Dan?
Mary:	(*after a moment*) Well…probably. I mean, I assume you asked us to do it for a reason.
Therapist:	Maybe it would be helpful to him, I don't know. There was only one way to find out! I think that is important to see here. That is, there might have been something of

value in that activity for Dan. Just as a moment ago there might have been something of value in learning more about what stops him—what stops all of us—from doing things we've committed to do. It may be that in "helping" him, you actually aligned with what might be keeping Dan—perhaps all of you—stuck.

Summary

We used this chapter to explore some of the issues therapists can encounter when doing group work, and how to work with those from within an ACT framework. Our greatest challenge while writing this chapter was keeping it from becoming a book in itself! As seasoned group therapists know all too well, there is no limit to what members (including ourselves) can bring to a session. We learned long ago to never say, "Now I've seen everything!"

In this chapter we demonstrated how applying ACT in a group setting offers the therapist a useful way to conceptualize whatever is occurring in session, including what's going on with individual members and with the group as a whole. The model consistently guides clinical decision making and helps therapists avoid some of the traps that can so easily occur in a group setting. It can help us even use clinical "missteps" to further the work. We have found that using ACT maximizes the therapeutic power of groups, harnessing what works and changing the function of what doesn't. When done well, it helps us bemused human beings reconcile with our basic natures while maximizing our lives. Good stuff!

PART 2

APPLYING ACT IN A GROUP SETTING

CHAPTER 4

Getting Started with an ACT Group

In this chapter we will set a framework for beginning an ACT group and learn how a therapist might plan for and initiate the first session. Over the next five chapters we will employ the same hypothetical group, utilizing discussion, exercises, sample dialogue, and commentary to demonstrate how to help group members build their skills with the core ACT processes. We will be speaking directly from our own experience and will also be taking you inside the mind of our hypothetical therapist to illustrate some of the clinical considerations and choice points that arise over the course of the therapy.

We do need to stress that our example group represents only one of many possible scenarios. For the purposes of instruction, this group has closed membership and meets on an outpatient basis for ninety minutes every week, for a total of twelve weeks. We used these criteria simply as a way to put shape to the group—to create a context for the following material. We could further specify, say, that group members have been referred by their primary care physician for treatment of depression, but these sorts of distinctions would not necessarily make this section more useful. Being based on universal principles of human behavior, ACT is transdiagnostic—the ideas and strategies put forth in the following pages should be applicable to a range of presenting problems. As you will see, a major thrust of this book is that working from within an ACT framework provides therapists with the means to effectively address the unique needs of their group members, regardless of presenting problem, history, or diagnosis. That said, other features, such as whether the group is ongoing or short term, whether membership is open or closed, or whether sessions last for an hour or several, do influence the overall approach, as we will address in chapter 11.

In this chapter, we will provide an overview of how to begin an ACT group. We will commence at a general level with some fundamental considerations and challenges that immediately arise from applying ACT as a model. We'll provide guidelines to help navigate these in a way that opens the path to psychological flexibility from the very start. We'll then review the overall objectives of an ACT group—the specific skills we would like to see group members develop and where we would like them to land at group's end. We will also cover the clinical tools we use to achieve these objectives, both within and outside of session. Next we'll move to basic approaches to the therapy, meaning how to introduce and move through the core processes so that group members have the opportunity to become adept at all six. We will then narrow our focus to specific session planning for this type of group, illustrating the considerations and decision making of our hypothetical therapist as she prepares for her first ACT group. This will include a discussion of when and how to target what unfolds in session. Finally, we will examine how fundamental tasks such as obtaining informed consent and establishing a supportive environment are viewed from the "ACT lens" and what this actually looks like in session.

In some ways we face a dilemma here similar to what a therapist encounters when starting an ACT group. That is, we anticipate that some of the ideas in this chapter won't "gel" until readers have a sense of how everything fits together. We believe the concepts introduced here will come together as we proceed through the book and ask that you bear with us as we move through uncertainty to a greater understanding of what this therapy is all about.

Inherent Challenges of the ACT Model

The very nature of ACT results in predictable tensions that are relevant the moment the therapy starts. These are not tensions that can be counteracted by establishing rules or defused by some upfront psychoeducation. Rather, the counterorthodox and counterintuitive characteristics of ACT must be held within the context of the group while the members (and even the therapist) adjust to new ways of being in group therapy. In this section we touch on these tensions and give some guidance as to how they can be navigated in a way that helps the group move forward.

ACT Is Counterorthodox

Historically, mental health treatment has been about fixing people, about making them "better." Our profession has striven for people to become psychologically healthy (i.e., not "ill" or "abnormal"), to think the right sorts of thoughts, to have the right sorts of feelings, to feel the right way about themselves and others. If this sounds judgmental, that is not our intention. This agenda is a product of languaging and is thus a human agenda. It is not surprising that our profession would align with the idea that this sort of fixing is the goal, or that the best way to help people is to get rid of the things that cause them pain.

The aim of ACT is quite different, however. Rather than align with a fix-me agenda, we work to help clients see what is already there. We help them recognize that they are already whole and acceptable, that they already have the capacity to live in the way they want to be living. Different histories, different memories, different thoughts, feelings, and sensations aren't required.

As nice as this might sound, it is not what most clients are seeking when they come to therapy. They want to feel better and are looking to the therapist for assistance in reaching that goal. This creates an inherent tension in the therapy from the moment it begins.

ACT Is Counterintuitive

On top of the fundamental dilemma just described, much of what is learned in ACT goes against the grain. For example, we humans put a lot of faith in our own minds. Thinking from (versus looking at) our thoughts is natural and easy, and we lack awareness of thinking as a process—as something we are doing. Accordingly, we treat the products of our minds as *the* reality, as literal truth. One of our favorite quotes, attributed to Emo Philips, says it all: "I used to think that the brain was the most wonderful organ in my body. Then I realized who was telling me this." In ACT we are after a different relationship with our minds—one that takes some getting used to.

This carries into other counterintuitive aspects of the therapy. For example, the idea that emotional pain or discomfort is in fact a part of living and not necessarily "wrong" is not what our minds tend to say! Simply letting internal discomfort *be* is truly a novel approach. Intentionally heading into discomfort (in the service of values) is not what we are used to doing.

It is also counterintuitive to hold our self-identities lightly, and yet that is a goal in ACT. We hope to help group members understand that they are more than the categorizations and evaluations they have learned to apply to themselves. This is a tough concept in itself, but especially tough when group members are invested in holding on to (or disproving) their identities for various reasons.

These are just a few of the ways in which ACT can run counter to what group members know, expect, and want, so starting on this journey will require a leap of faith. Group members have yet to learn how the model applies to their lives and what it might offer. In fact, understanding the benefits of ACT requires the very skills we hope to develop in the therapy. Let's turn to how we can help our group take this leap of faith.

Navigating Challenges from Within the Model

Paradoxically, the same tenets that make ACT somewhat challenging can effectively be used to work through those challenges. That is, by holding to the model, the therapist is guided to approach some of these tensions in a way that actually helps members progress. Here are some guidelines we have found particularly helpful:

Remember this tension doesn't have to be resolved. As ACT therapists, we are presented with an opportunity to walk the walk the moment we begin the therapy. We are using this model with the belief that it will help group members get unstuck and engaged in vital, meaningful living; we understand the route we plan to take and why we take that route. Group members do not have this knowledge, and uncertainty, confusion, and ambivalence are understandable responses to being in that place. This situation does not need to be fixed or resolved, so much as noticed and held.

> *Therapist:* A funny thing about this therapy is that it involves an approach to life that can seem *really* different, maybe completely foreign. In my experience it can take a while before it starts to makes sense. Some pieces need to come together first. Until that happens it's likely we'll experience all sorts of things in here: confusion, uncertainty…even frustration. So our first challenge, our task, is to make room for that stuff to be there while we proceed down this path. It's a natural part of the experience and doesn't need to be gone in order for us to move forward.

Here the therapist has normalized what the group is likely to experience during the course of therapy. She is already working within the model by pointing the way to how such experiences might usefully be held.

Aim for transparency. In ACT we draw upon the notion of therapist transparency again and again. By transparency, we refer to being present and open to our experience in the group and using this to model the abilities targeted in the therapy. At the start of an ACT group, therapist transparency helps establish a culture that is ACT-consistent. It also allows the therapist to acknowledge the tensions we have been discussing, without aligning with what has kept members stuck.

> *Therapist:* I'm noticing what's coming up for me right now. On the one hand I feel excited about this group. I'm excited about doing ACT with you all and can't wait to get going. On the other, I'm worried about what you will think of it, whether you will like it—all that stuff. I notice a pull to try to fix all that, an urge to tell you everything I can about the therapy and convince you that it's great…but I think it's important to let all that stuff be in the room. Wherever you are with this, wherever *I* am with this, is okay. We don't need to feel any different or have different thoughts going on; we can take it all with us as we head in.

Create space for something new. There's no denying it takes a bit of skill to move the group forward within a cultural context that runs counter to the model. We create space for new learning by meeting our group members with compassion and understanding, while at the same time pointing to where we are headed in the therapy. In chapter 1 we talked about the importance of how we as therapists show up in the room. If we can remember we are in the same struggle as our group members—the struggle of being human—we are helped to remain humble and respectful of how they experience things. By requiring of ourselves what we will require of the group (walking the walk), we show the way. We will provide many examples of this in the following chapters.

Don't align. It can be helpful to remember that choosing not to do something can be an effective intervention. Though time is needed for group members to develop psychological flexibility, we can open the door by making sure not to align with the processes that lead to psychological inflexibility. For example, in an initial session you can expect to see a lot of fusion with thoughts and rules and a lot of strategies aimed toward avoiding or reducing discomfort. In fact, we're willing to bet you will see these in yourself! This is a clinical opportunity. If you can recognize these processes as they arise, you can respond in a way that furthers the work.

> *Mary:*   I'm really anxious about this group… I've done groups before and they just don't work for me. (*to therapist*) How do I know this is going to be any different?

> *Therapist:*   (*nodding empathetically and gently smiling*) Yeah! (*sits*)

Of course a therapist could respond to Mary's comment in any number of ways. If we focus on ACT processes, however, we are guided as to what we might *not* want to do. For starters, we could hypothesize that Mary is fused with thoughts and experientially avoidant—she seems to be looking to the therapist for a way out of what she is experiencing in the moment. Rather than align with that agenda by attempting to answer Mary's questions or otherwise assuage her concerns, our therapist modeled willingness. There is a quietly potent message in there: *We can handle this.* The therapist also modeled defusion—defusing from *Mary's* thoughts (and probably her own) that Mary's question must be answered. Though subtle, this intervention can really pack a punch as it is likely radically different from what Mary is used to. The function of her question (e.g., we hypothesize that Mary is trying to fix feelings of anxiety and fears about the future by seeking a guarantee) didn't work as she intended. (Note that the function of this particular intervention also depends on its consequences. That is, if the therapist's simple "Yeah" led to Mary also sitting with what she was experiencing a bit, perhaps starting to ask a question and then stopping, it could be hypothesized that it "worked" as intended. However, if Mary immediately launched into even more questions, we could hypothesize that it did not. Tracking how interventions function will help the therapist determine what to do next.)

Be patient. It is helpful to remember that this is a process and that there will be many opportunities to work with the core processes at the heart of ACT. Not everything has to be resolved all at once; there isn't just one moment of opportunity we must seize. This allows us to be patient, to meet the group where it is while filing away something to address at a later point in time.

Building Psychological Flexibility in a Group

We stated in chapter 1 that the overarching aim in ACT is psychological flexibility, and we now turn to how we go about achieving this in a group setting. We will examine how an ACT therapist utilizes a combination of psychoeducation and direct experiences both in and outside of session to help group members develop and then usefully apply those skills that constitute psychological flexibility.

Perhaps the simplest way to phrase what we aim for in the group is helping members get unstuck and moving in their lives, meaning living in a way that is vital and meaningful according to each group member. This requires identifying and clarifying personal values and learning to make choices in accordance with those values—moving from unworkable behaviors to those that further who they want to be and how they want to be living. There is a lot packed into that simple idea! Unworkable behaviors are often about trying to escape, avoid, or otherwise control unwanted (e.g., uncomfortable, painful) thoughts, feelings, and physical sensations. Sometimes, what's not working is waiting for the "right" sort of thoughts and feelings to show up before one starts living, such as waiting for "confidence" or "motivation" or going for immediate gratification despite significant costs, as with a gambling addiction. So the aim is helping the group members recognize that these sorts of agendas are unsuccessful and/or too costly and learn to relate to their internal experiences in a different way.

Again, that simple idea involves several key abilities. Members will need to be able to bring their awareness to what they are actually experiencing and doing in the present moment. This will require some degree of willingness to have what is there to be experienced, and the ability to "get out of one's head" enough to track what is going on and to perceive thoughts as only a part of that reality. It will be important for them to understand that thoughts don't necessarily represent "truth" and that one can notice a thought without being slave to it. In essence, group members will need to build awareness of the distinction between the thoughts, feelings, and sensations of the moment—the internal experiences—and the self, the Experiencer that can notice and simply hold those experiences. These abilities enable them to make value-driven choices, to get going in their lives *now*.

In order to help group members build psychological flexibility, we rely both on psychoeducation and direct experience. As we move through each process in the upcoming chapters, we will highlight the concepts that are conveyed to the group by teaching. We will also provide numerous examples of experiential work that provides opportunities for group members to practice the abilities that are the focus of the therapy.

Psychoeducation

A funny thing about ACT is that although the therapy was derived as a way to redress problematic effects of languaging, we rely upon language to do the work! In fact, the same language processes that lead to human suffering are used to free clients from that suffering. Throughout this book we will demonstrate how we use language very deliberately in ACT—we try to undermine language processes that work against psychological flexibility while strengthening those that benefit group members in some way.

We rely on discourse as a way to impart new ideas, point to things, and elicit and reinforce the behaviors that produce meaningful change. Each of the behavioral processes targeted in ACT involves key concepts that can facilitate growth when grasped at an intellectual level. As we move through each process in the pages that follow, we will highlight the ideas we consider central to each and provide examples as to how we might explicitly explore these with the group.

Our theoretical roots guide us to be wary of words, however, and we draw strongly upon experiential learning in our sessions. It is often the case that direct experience can accomplish what words cannot, and it is safe to say that intellectual understanding is not what this therapy is about. It's about "moving with your feet," and we want to provide ample opportunity for this as the therapy unfolds.

Direct Experience

By direct experience we refer to nonverbal learning and experiencing. This can be deliberately invoked (e.g., conducting an experiential exercise) or pointed out as it naturally occurs (e.g., guiding group members to contact what they are feeling). It would be erroneous to imply that these sorts of activities are purely experiential. They entail language processes as well—whether as instructions to set up an exercise or direct attention, to internally assess and process an experience, or as the rationale for how one responds. The interventions mentioned below share the common feature of not simply relying on the exchange of verbal information, but pulling for a felt *experience* in the room:

Contacting the present: It can be said that experiential learning is always going on, whether or not we are aware of it. For example, an individual experiencing panic symptoms might not be aware that she is linking those symptoms to the context in which they are occurring, or that she is reinforcing those symptoms by escaping, but nonetheless those associations are made. We are always experiencing and learning by that experiencing. In ACT, we aim to capitalize on this learning by bringing awareness to it and by creating opportunities for experiential learning to occur.

There are two main reasons for this. One is that when group members are better able to attend to what they are experiencing—what they are doing, feeling, thinking, and sensing—they have greater access to the information that is available in the moment. For example, the individual experiencing panic can also notice that she is actually safe, that she is not being threatened even though her mind is full of thoughts about being unsafe and needing to escape.

This touches on the second, related reason for bringing awareness to the present moment. When we contact the present more fully, that is, get out of our minds and into the moment, whatever's going on in our minds has less influence. It becomes only part of what we are experiencing at any given time. So despite a slew of furious thoughts about what his child has done wrong, an angry father could look in his child's eyes, take a breath, and engage calmly. The individual with panic could opt to stay in the anxiety-provoking situation and see what happens next.

In-the-moment interventions: The above discussion explains why we prioritize in-the-moment learning in ACT. That is, if the therapist is engaged in teaching the group about an ACT concept, and then something occurs in group that actually demonstrates that concept, the therapist would likely direct attention to that in-the-moment experience. Or, if a discussion isn't going anywhere, rather than try harder with words, the therapist might turn to an experiential exercise as an alternate learning modality. If something is happening in the group that is distracting or otherwise functioning as a barrier to learning, the therapist would work with that in-the-moment experience (we provided examples of this in chapter 3). Again, direct observation, experiential awareness, and doing can often accomplish what talking cannot.

Experiential exercises: The problematic effects of languaging lead us to turn to experiential exercises as a means to develop the skills targeted in ACT. We use this term to refer to therapist-led activities specifically designed to illuminate one or more ACT processes. They can be used to increase an ability such as willingness or defusion, to demonstrate ways in which members get stuck, or to pull the core processes together. There are numerous examples of experiential exercises in the ACT literature, and each of the forthcoming applied chapters (see also Supplemental Exercises at http://www.newharbin ger.com/23994) provides examples we have found useful in a group setting.

Modeling: An ACT therapist will often model how to contact (experience) the moment and share how she is experiencing the group as a way to further the therapy. One of the most effective ways of learning is by observation, and therapists can greatly facilitate learning by modeling the abilities they are hoping to develop in the group.

This is not restricted to therapist modeling, however. One of the strengths of group work is that members learn from one another's behavior, both what is useful and what is not so useful. A skilled therapist is adept at flushing out examples of both as they arise in session.

Of course, modeling as an intervention is not unique to ACT. The principles forming ACT specifically guide *what* is being modeled, however, which we will discuss at length in the following pages. We will also explore when modeling might be augmented by discussing it explicitly (e.g., "Mary, I'm appreciating how you resisted the urge just then to rescue Dan") or when it might be more powerful to allow an experience to sit without words getting in the way (e.g., the therapist simply sits silently as a way to help the group members contact their feelings).

Promoting Growth Outside of Session

We have been discussing ways to promote learning within the group. Now we turn to how we help members continue their learning between sessions and, most importantly, apply that learning to their daily lives.

Homework: An ACT therapist will often assign tasks designed to build skills between sessions, such as asking members to practice mindfulness for a few minutes every day. We might assign homework that engages core processes and helps move the therapy along, such as asking the group to complete a values worksheet before the next session. Because the term "homework" can bring up unhelpful associations for some members, we often phrase between-session tasks as "practice" or as "committed actions." In chapter 10 we will discuss ways to address problems that can arise with assigning homework, such as how to work with group members who do not complete agreed-upon tasks.

Translation: One of the most effective ways to help group members apply what they are learning in ACT is by helping them see how the core processes manifest in their daily lives. Just as we help group members understand the ways in which they keep themselves stuck, we also point to ways they are already employing the abilities targeted in ACT. For example, the therapist might ask the group whether anyone felt like sleeping a bit later that day (typically most will quickly say yes). He might then point out that despite thoughts and feelings about wanting to sleep more, they nonetheless got out of bed.

Remembering that the skills that make up psychological flexibility are on a continuum, we help members see how deficits in certain areas play out in their lives. For example, early on we might ask the group members to track the various ways they attempt to control unwanted thoughts or feelings during the week. This could increase awareness of the unworkability of this strategy, paving the way to choose willingness as an alternative. Or we might ask members to work on noticing their thoughts as they go about their lives, which not only helps them notice how often they are thinking from (rather than looking at) their thoughts, but might also help them develop the ability to defuse from thoughts.

Committed actions: A strength of group therapy is the opportunity it offers for members to support one another's growth. The universality of the processes targeted in ACT enhances that sort of you-me translation. As one member works through a challenging situation, the others can see how the same processes play out in their own lives and what they might do differently. Just as group members can enable dysfunctional ways of being in the world, so too can social support facilitate actions that are in line with how members actually want to be living. In ACT we harness this social force by helping group members articulate personal values and then verbalize discrete actions they can take in accordance with those values.

The term "bold move" is often used in ACT to denote a type of committed action. Like committed actions, a bold move is deliberately chosen and value driven. "Bold" is used as an invitation, the emphasis being on what might be challenging as opposed to what might feel safe or easiest. In being bold, these behavioral commitments necessarily involve all of the core processes in ACT. The individual must be willing to have whatever shows up in taking this action and have the ability to see uncomfortable thoughts, feelings, and sensations for what they are. That requires something larger than all that stuff, something that pulls them forward (i.e., values). This doesn't mean a bold move must entail going to Antarctica to save the penguins—it can be something quiet, such as attending that art class, or making that phone call. What is "bold" differs from individual to individual, but the idea is that whatever the action, it requires some willingness and committed action to see it through.

Charting a Course for an ACT Group

We have laid out the specific skills we hope to build in an ACT group and the means we use to develop those abilities. But how do we actually proceed? When do we introduce willingness, for example? When is it time to work on defusion? When do we begin to explore values? In actuality, the ubiquity and interrelatedness of the core processes means there are all sorts of opportunities to work with them. At any given moment one could focus on contacting the present, on willingness to have one's experience, on defusion, on choosing a committed action, and so on.

That said, some concepts and abilities are easier to grasp than others, and understanding and increasing skill with one core process can pave the way for another. For this reason, when the setting and type of group allows, it is common to move through the central domains of ACT in a sequential fashion, and we will demonstrate that method in the next six chapters. We have found this approach more accessible for therapists newer to the therapy, and it also ensures that all the key ACT processes are well covered. We have discovered, however, that therapists typically become more and more "fluid" in their approach to the therapy as their familiarity with it grows, being able to move smoothly from one process to another, pulling out and working with whatever has shown up in the room or seems to need attention. The more therapists can recognize and work flexibly with the core processes as they arise, the more sensitive they can be to what is unfolding in that moment with their particular clients.

For the purposes of this book, we have chosen to demonstrate a sequence that reflects the behavioral pillars described in chapter 1. That is, the processes targeted in ACT can be parsed into three main behavioral pillars (Hayes et al., 1999): open (willing and defused), centered (present and aware of self-as-context), and engaged (values and committed action), and our hypothetical group will move through the therapy in that order.

Clinical Considerations in Planning for an ACT Group

In the next several chapters we will demonstrate how to go about treatment planning for an ACT group. As mentioned, we will use a hypothetical therapist working with a particular type of group (twelve week outpatient group with closed membership), which will influence these decisions. In chapter 11 we will address treatment planning for other types of groups; however, readers will likely gain insights into other group formats as we examine the clinical considerations that pertain to this particular sort of group below.

Open versus closed membership: Since this group will have closed membership, the therapist will not need to accommodate individuals who are entering the group at different times. A sequential approach to the therapy will work well with this type of group.

Inpatient versus outpatient: The fact that this group will meet once per week on an outpatient basis has a couple of clinical implications. One is that participants seem to be functioning well enough in their lives that they do not require more intensive treatment. Another is that they will spend a lot of time between sessions in contexts that may not support, or that may even work against, the therapy. Earlier we referred to the counterintuitive nature of ACT; in fact, many ACT tenets run counter to our culture (e.g., we live in a culture that promotes a control agenda). Furthermore, in order to apply what they are learning in the group to their lives, group members will be tasked to respond in new ways to very old phenomena. This suggests our therapist will need to assign between-session tasks or practice that will help the group swim up this stream. It also suggests that members might need some reorienting when they return to group, such as a recap of the main points covered and what they have learned so far. The therapist will need to draw a thread through the core processes so that as the group moves through them, members will be able to understand both how the processes relate to one another and how they apply to their daily lives.

Session length: This group will meet for ninety minutes every week, which should allow the therapist plenty of time for discussion and at least one or two experiential exercises per group.

Length of therapy: Our hypothetical group will meet for twelve sessions, so our therapist knows she has adequate time to work sequentially through the six core processes. She expects to spend more time on some processes than others depending on how her group responds. For example, she anticipates moving fairly quickly through contacting the present as she has found that members typically grasp this concept rather easily (though the *ability* to contact the present will need to be developed throughout the therapy). She has found that self-as-context is usually harder for folks, so she anticipates needing more sessions to work on that piece. She also wants to make sure there is plenty of time for members to practice applying what they have learned in the group, so she plans to have a couple of sessions for this after all the processes have been worked through and are in play. Below is a rough timeline she developed for her group—rough because what actually unfolds in session will trump any planned agenda. (We will list only session topics here, as the following chapters will cover each of these in detail.)

Pillar One—Open (ACT processes: willingness and defusion)

    Session 1: Housekeeping, Group Culture, Conceptualization, Creative Hopelessness

    Session 2: Control as the Problem/Willingness

    Session 3: Willingness/Defusion

    Session 4: Defusion

Pillar Two—Centered (ACT processes: contacting the present, self-as-context)

    Session 5: Contacting the Present

    Session 6: Self-as-Context

    Session 7: Self-as-Context

Pillar Three—Engaged (ACT processes: values and committed action)

    Session 8: Values

    Session 9: Values

    Session 10: Committed Action

    Session 11: Pulling it all together

    Session 12: Pulling it all together

Planning for Session 1

As she thinks about her initial ACT session, our therapist considers four main objectives: (1) completing fundamental tasks such as obtaining informed consent, reviewing group logistics (e.g., when and where to meet, any attendance requirements, how to communicate if needed between sessions), discussing confidentiality, and setting expectations for participation; (2) beginning to establish a group culture that is conducive to growth and is ACT-consistent; (3) developing an initial conceptualization of her group members from within an ACT framework; and (4) beginning the work of developing psychological flexibility. Let's take a closer look at each of these topics:

1. Housekeeping: Our therapist is aware she needs to complete the fundamental tasks mentioned above and will incorporate these in her first session. (We anticipate readers will be familiar with such tasks. The model does have implications for how our therapist goes about these tasks, however, and we provide detailed examples later in this chapter.)

2. Group culture: We have already pointed to ways in which the therapist's approach to this initial session can open the door to psychological flexibility. Shortly we will demonstrate how she will use even basic tasks to further the work.

3. Conceptualization: Our therapist has gathered information on individual group members from an initial intake. She therefore has some sense of who is in the group, but she fully expects to refine that assessment as the group unfolds. She wants to develop an ACT conceptualization of her group members, meaning where they are in terms of the core ACT processes (e.g., willingness or avoidance, contacting the present or being fused with thoughts, self-as-context or rigid attachment to a conceptualized self, clearly defined values or lack thereof, and level of committed action). In this initial session she wants to learn how her members experience their world and themselves as well as what they feel is missing or not working in their lives.

4. Creative hopelessness: The therapist wants to waste no time in moving toward psychological flexibility. This means flushing out and challenging unworkable agendas group members are likely bringing to the therapy, such as wanting to be "fixed." At the same time, she is cognizant of how teaching/telling/persuading would likely backfire and therefore plans to proceed in a way that validates each member's experience while also gently illuminating the predicament each is in (i.e., trying to fix or control what can't be fixed or controlled). The idea is to engender an experience of "creative hopelessness" (Hayes et al., 2011), wherein members recognize that what they've been attempting hasn't worked (and doesn't work), thereby making space to learn something new.

Session Strategy. Our therapist has developed the following plan for her first group session: She will start off by welcoming members and having them introduce themselves to one another. She will discuss group logistics, participation expectations, and other housekeeping tasks, including limits of confidentiality and informed consent. Next she will engage the group in a process known as "creative hopelessness" (detailed in the following chapter). This procedure provides a great deal of information: what members perceive as the problem, how they have dealt with it, and where they have gotten stuck. It is geared toward drawing out the control or fix-me agenda, placing it squarely on the table as unworkable.

In this first session, our therapist is not aiming for group members to suddenly shift into willingness or give up the control agenda; this is the work of the therapeutic process that has yet to unfold. Rather, she simply wants to highlight the bind of the struggle itself as a means to create an opening for something new.

Near the end of the discussion, our therapist plans to introduce an ACT metaphor, the man in a hole (Hayes et al., 1999), to further highlight the dilemma of pursuing a strategy that doesn't work. She does not want to introduce other core processes or do anything that will take away from what she has developed in the session, and she wants her group to start learning how to "simply sit" with something. She will conclude by assigning homework: she'll ask members to notice a situation in which they are trying to apply control, and have the willingness to have that experience, to sit with it.

Now that we've explored decisions involved in planning for session 1, let's look more broadly at decision making as it applies to all sessions.

Guidelines for Approaching Clinical Decision Making in ACT

As any group therapist will tell you (and as you have probably experienced), having a planned agenda only goes so far. Along with determining how to proceed through the core processes and developing session plans, there is the small matter of what actually happens in session. Because the core ACT processes run through everything that occurs in session, it can be challenging to determine what to focus on and how best to do so. Is it time to offer some psychoeducation, or would it be more effective to move straight to an experiential exercise? Does it make sense to respond directly to a question raised by someone in the group, or would it be better to direct attention to the present? Should you explore values because a group member made a remark that pointed to that process, or should you stick with working on defusion as planned? These decisions depend on context, including what's going on with a particular group member, what's going on with the group as a whole, and what's going on with the therapy overall. The following guidelines will help you in making these decisions:

It's not about the content. One of the most central implications of using ACT as a model is its emphasis on function over form. That is, it's not the form (we could also say "content") of the thoughts, nor the type (we could also say "form") of emotion or sensation that can cause problems; rather, it's how those internal experiences function for the individual. A group member could have many thoughts about wanting to die, but the thoughts themselves don't do damage. What can be problematic is how those thoughts influence the individual's behavior, or in other words, how those thoughts function. The group member with anxiety could spend years upon years trying not to have worrisome thoughts, or the emotion of fear, or the physical sensations of anxiety—or she could relate to those thoughts, feelings, and sensations in a way that allows her to live her life.

Focusing on the process rather than the content is another way to talk about this. That is, in ACT we look to see how the processes targeted in the model manifest in the session and in group members' lives. So when group members comment, or raise a question, or share an experience, or respond non-verbally (e.g., shrug, frown, laugh, tune out), the therapist looks to see what core process(es) might be in play. Although this takes some practice, once you learn to recognize core processes as they arise in session, you are able to further the therapy regardless of what members bring to the table. You are also freed from trying to resolve or fix things that can't be fixed. Let's use an example to demonstrate this as well as some other clinical considerations we will be discussing in this section.

A group member announced that her weekend was ruined because her mother-in-law came to visit and was "critical as usual." This sort of comment pulls for a content-level response, such as, "I'm sorry to hear that! What did she say?" While such a response might feel validating to the group member, it doesn't enable her to deal with this situation in a more workable way. Viewing this remark through that ACT lens, however, we might hypothesize that the group member is fused with some verbal rules around what weekends are supposed to look like, how mothers-in-law are supposed to act, what it means if one is criticized, and so on. We might note how the group member is relating to her internal experiences—that because she was having certain thoughts and feelings, her weekend was ruined. This again suggests fusion with the belief that she cannot have a more satisfactory weekend if she is experiencing those thoughts and feelings, and a lack of willingness and self-as-context.

To continue, we can surmise that being criticized is painful for this group member, which points to problematic attachment to a conceptualized self. In other words, she may believe she either is or is not okay depending on what others think of her. This again suggests fusion with thoughts and a deficit in experiencing self-as-context. There are more possibilities here, but we can see how this hypothesizing orients the therapist to what might be keeping this group member stuck. It is not her mother-in-law, as difficult as she may be. Rather, when her mother-in-law is critical, this group member experiences a set of thoughts, feelings, and sensations that then influence her own behavior such that her weekend is "ruined." She would likely benefit from learning to contact the present and defuse from thoughts, from recognizing that she is actually intact and larger than the painful thoughts and feelings that come up when criticized (to experience self-as-context), and from learning to make choices that take her in the direction of her values despite unpleasant thoughts and feelings (willingness, values, and committed action).

Ultimately, we aim to be working primarily with function rather than content. That is, we hope that the focus of the group will be on how members can live vitally and well regardless of—or along with—the thoughts, feelings, and sensations that show up as a part of living. Of course, thoughts and feelings matter, but they are treated as experiences to be had while focusing on moving forward in a valued direction.

Consider timing. Clinical timing in ACT requires a consideration of the group's understanding and skill level with the core ACT processes at any given point in the therapy. Have group members just been introduced to a process or have they developed some ability with it? Is a group member demonstrating a particular deficit that needs to be addressed before moving on? Is it time to pull everything together? In considering timing, we also think about the nature of what is being taught. Is it complex? Is it something that could use some initial psychoeducation, or does it lend itself better to an exercise than to words?

As an example, the ability to contact the present requires some degree of willingness and some ability to defuse from thoughts. It also involves experiencing self-as-context—all skills we hope to develop in the therapy. Initially, however, inviting the group to simply sit quietly for a few moments and notice whatever is coming up for them (i.e., building the core processes of contacting the present and willingness) might be a big enough challenge. Once this sort of holding and noticing has been established, the therapist could expand this to learning to notice and defuse from thoughts, and ultimately to "noticing the Noticer" (i.e., to experience self-as-context).

Let's continue with the mother-in-law example to demonstrate how timing considerations guide intervention decisions. If this group member made the comment about her mother-in-law near the beginning of the therapy, for example, we might choose to highlight what hasn't worked. For instance, the therapist might ask the group member what sorts of things she's tried to avoid feeling the way she does when criticized by her mother-in-law. This intervention is designed to undermine a problematic control agenda—that the group member's mother-in-law, or more accurately, the thoughts and feelings our group member has around her mother-in-law—need to be somehow fixed.

Perhaps the therapist has been working with this group for a bit and has noticed this member has consistent difficulty being in the present. In that case the therapist might take this opportunity to develop that skill, asking the group member to shift her attention from the story about her mother-in-law to what she is experiencing in the moment as she talks about it with the group. If the group as a whole has been learning about defusing from thoughts, the therapist could ask the group member to track the thoughts that showed up as the situation with her mother-in-law was unfolding. She could then extend that to the present moment, asking her what thoughts are showing up for her in the moment, and asking other group members what thoughts they are noticing as well. If the group has been nearing the end of the therapy (i.e., all the core ACT processes had been introduced and developed to some degree), the therapist might simply ask, "Given this situation with your mother-in-law, what might you have done last weekend that took you in the direction of your values?"

Consider explicit versus nonexplicit interventions. Particularly when conducting ACT in a sequential fashion, therapists can be thrown when something occurs in session that points to a process that has yet to be introduced to the group. For example, a group member could respond in a way that strongly suggests learning to experience self-as-context would be beneficial, but the therapist hadn't planned on introducing that process to the group for a few sessions yet. Also, because the processes are interrelated, it is likely that several are in play at any given moment even though the therapist is ostensibly focusing on just one.

Considering the distinction between explicit and nonexplicit work can be helpful here. By explicit work we simply mean the therapist specifically refers to the particular process she is focusing on, such as "willingness" or "defusing" from thoughts (or "observing thoughts"—the exact wording isn't the point, just that the process itself is being explicitly discussed). In contrast, we loosely use the term "nonexplicit" to refer to the technique of furthering a process without specifically discussing it.

As you will see in the following pages, we use nonexplicit methods to help group members build facility with core ACT processes right from the start of therapy. We seek opportunities to work with what naturally arises in session, utilizing language, modeling, and in-the-moment experiential work to further the abilities of both individual members and the group as a whole. Having these methods at our disposal means we don't have to forgo addressing something that has shown up in the moment. We can work with it indirectly while waiting to address it explicitly with the group when it seems best to do so.

When it is time to explore a process explicitly, we typically introduce the topic to the group and generate a discussion, meanwhile continuing to work with present-moment examples as they arise in session. We might determine that it would be most productive to introduce a new concept to the group in a very concrete, linear way, for example, "Today I'd like to explore the idea of how control can actually keep us stuck." At other times, we might decide that moving into an exercise without prior explanation could lead to a more impactful learning experience—one in which group members are provided an opportunity to have their own aha moment. We would then engage the group in a discussion following the exercise, making sure the central points were conveyed.

As you can see, there is no overarching algorithm here; the skill is about taking contextual variables into consideration and making the best move one can. As we walk through an application of ACT in chapters 5 through 10, we will demonstrate how we navigate some of these choice points during the course of the therapy.

Remember the point of talking. In keeping the overarching objective of ACT front and center, the ACT therapist is guided to use talking as a means to develop the skills that increase psychological flexibility. The point isn't that the group members understand what defusion is, for example, but that they learn to defuse from their thoughts. We don't want them to merely understand what is meant by self-as-context, but to be able to contact that sort of self-experiencing in any given moment. Words are used to help these key abilities along—by introducing them conceptually, by pointing them out as they arise in the therapy, and by guiding the group to engage in activities that provide opportunities for practice. Keeping this in mind helps the therapist notice when he is talking at the cost of doing. It helps him remember to look for in-the-moment examples of what he is trying to convey, and to pull in experiential exercises that will provide opportunities for the group to directly experience and practice what he is wanting them to learn.

Include experiential exercises in every session. We do make sure that every group session contains some experiential work. One way to ensure this happens is to plan a structured experiential exercise or two that demonstrates what will be covered in the group. In the following applied chapters, and in the accompanying online content, we will provide numerous examples of exercises that do this nicely. We have observed, however, that as therapists become more facile with the therapy, they are able to devise novel exercises on the fly based on what is unfolding in session. In fact, this phenomenon is one of the reasons there is an ever-expanding number of exercises available in the ACT literature.

Be present. A common feature of all these guidelines is that they require the therapist be present in the session. Though the therapist may have a plan for the session, he remains present to what is actually unfolding in the group. He may work with something on a content level, such as responding to a question, while also attending to how that question is currently functioning. He might be midstream with an experiential exercise, but being present to the moment he can recognize if it isn't working and respond accordingly. He can recognize and work with the core ACT processes that arise during the session. Most importantly, he is present to his own experience in the group—he's able to use that as a source of information and, through modeling, as a means of furthering the therapy.

Completing Essential Tasks from Within an ACT Framework

We imagine most of our readers are familiar with initial session tasks such as obtaining informed consent and discussing confidentiality. However, even these fundamental tasks take on additional nuances when viewed through the ACT lens, and we'll now turn to how to approach these tasks within an ACT framework. We will then wrap up this chapter by giving readers a sense of what an ACT group looks like in the room.

Informed Consent

It's worth noting here that many therapists report that obtaining informed consent in ACT can be surprisingly hard. It is challenging to adequately convey what ACT is about when that understanding requires some additional learning and skill development. One helpful hint is to not attempt to "tell" the group the whole gist of ACT by stating, for example, "In this group you will learn to accept difficult thoughts and feelings and to defuse from what your mind is telling you so that you can make choices according to what you value." First, it is unlikely the group will understand what is meant by such a summary or how these principles might personally apply. The result is that this sort of introduction doesn't actually function as a means of obtaining informed consent. Second, terms such as "acceptance" and "values" can be pretty loaded. Members often make immediate assumptions based upon their own learning histories with these terms that actually run counter to the therapy. Third, because we are operating from within an ACT framework, we are wary of the mind's tendency to want everything spelled out and neatly wrapped up—God forbid we venture into the unknown! Finally, ACT is a present-focused, highly experiential therapy. Every group, indeed every member, will have its own unique experience as it unfolds. With all this said, as mental health providers we are required to obtain informed consent and agree that group members need to know what they are signing up for. What to do?

As we will see repeatedly throughout the next few chapters, being authentically present and transparent offers a way through such dilemmas.

> *Therapist:* I find that trying to inform people about ACT can be sort of tricky. That is, you have a right to understand what this therapy is about, and at the same time, it's hard to know what our experience as a group will be. Each group is different. I can say that this therapy is about engaging in life in a vital way and that this group will be like that as well. You will feel things in here. This therapy can also be very different from other therapies you may have encountered. We will be working on a particular approach to living, one that offers a way to live in an engaged and meaningful way, even if tough things are going on. Since it takes a few sessions for things to come together so that you can experience this for yourselves, I'm asking that you hang in there for maybe three or four sessions—enough time to get a sense of the therapy. We can then check in and see how you feel it's going. Would that be an acceptable way to go?

Here the therapist is inviting the group to hold the inherent ambiguity that comes from heading into the unknown (willingness), while also demonstrating understanding and respect for members' experiences.

Protecting Confidentiality

A subtle difference in how an ACT therapist might approach confidentiality is how the inherent problem of privacy in a group setting is held. That is, the therapist simply cannot guarantee confidentiality in a group—it is an aspect of group therapy that cannot be fixed. Group members must then participate "in good faith," understanding that they cannot be sure what they share will stay in the room (requiring willingness, defusion, values, committed action). The therapist acknowledges this problem and can certainly attempt to raise the odds that members will respect one another's privacy. At the same time, she models simply holding this sort of ambiguity while moving forward.

Therapist: One of the things we really try to protect in therapy is patient (client) confidentiality. In a group like this, where there are many participants, I do not have the ability to guarantee that what happens in here will remain confidential. We all take a bit of a leap of faith in here, taking the chance to participate anyway in order to get something out of this process. We each have the ability to take the risk, and we each have the ability to protect the confidentiality of this group. I can certainly commit to that. Would you all be willing to make a commitment that you will not share what happens in this group elsewhere?

This verbal commitment can be emphasized by having all members, one by one, state their commitment to keeping the group process confidential.

Establishing a Safe and Supportive Environment

Let's start with looking at what is typically meant by a "safe and supportive" group. It might mean a group where certain behaviors (e.g., ridiculing, shaming) are not tolerated, or one in which confidentiality is protected. These sorts of guidelines make sense and are doable. There is another notion of safe and supportive that is not so doable, however. That is, when group members (and often therapists) speak of wanting a group to be "safe," what they often are seeking is *emotional* safety. They want to know that members will not be emotionally hurt in the group. Ensuring this sort of safety is not possible, nor is it desirable.

One of the tenets of ACT is that trying to control our internal experiences just doesn't work in general. Whether we're striving to feel at ease in a group, working to avoid embarrassment or anxiety, or aiming for happiness like some sort of destination, it is this very agenda that can cause us to become stuck. A major goal of the therapy is to help members learn they can experience what is there to be had internally while *doing* what works (e.g., participating in the group). As we will see in the following pages, we also work to help group members contact a self that is intact, regardless of the thoughts and feelings going on. When we align with the idea that members are so fragile that they are destroyed somehow by painful thoughts or feelings, we are directly contradicting the tenets of ACT.

This is an important paradox to see, as seeking some guarantee of emotional safety can function as a real barrier to participation: "I'm not going to share because I don't feel safe," or, "You have to prove that you're safe before I can trust you with my stuff." Even more importantly, holding this idea of emotional safety out as a goal supports the notion that someone is not okay if he is feeling hurt, anxious, judged, or otherwise uncomfortable in group.

For this reason an ACT therapist is unlikely to say something like "It is important that everyone feels safe in this group." Rather, we might emphasize doable behaviors by stating, "It is important that we treat each other with respect. That might look like doing our best to listen to one another, to offer feedback in a way that is courteous…" We look for opportunities to reinforce behaviors that facilitate the group process while refraining from supporting the idea that members are fragile. For example, the therapist might remark, "I think it's really cool that you just shared that even though you seemed a little worried about what the group would think," rather than, "I'm glad you know you are safe enough in this group to share that."

Physical Setup

To wrap up this chapter on getting started in ACT, we'll give you a quick picture of how we physically set up an ACT group. We prefer to conduct the therapy in a circle. This facilitates intimacy and engagement and reflects the idea that each individual—including the therapist—is an equal participant. We typically have a whiteboard nearby for use as needed. Some of the experiential exercises use props, so if we anticipate conducting one of those exercises in the group, we will have the required articles standing by.

Although we suppose the above description does not differ much from other therapy groups, a potential difference with ACT is the emphasis on being present in the group. We discourage group members from reading things or taking notes in session, preferring they just be present to what's happening in the room. We assure them there will be ample opportunities to learn the key concepts as we will be revisiting them repeatedly throughout the therapy. We do provide handouts if appropriate and follow up with written work such as values worksheets. In general, though, we do not want a bunch of papers functioning as a barrier to experience. This applies to the therapist as well; we would argue that an imperfect delivery of an exercise by a therapist who is authentically present to the group is preferable to one flawlessly read from a script. We look for any means to create the same sort of group experience we are hoping members will learn to create in their lives: authentic connection, living in the present, and vital engagement in life according to personal values.

Furthering ACT with Basic Tasks

Once the essential tasks are completed, it's time to head into the therapy. We must stress, however, that the work in ACT has already begun. That is, rather than attempt to spell out what the group will experience in ACT, the therapist has pointed to the ambiguity inherent in the therapeutic process, suggesting this be simply acknowledged and held for a bit. This draws upon the core processes of being present, willingness/acceptance, and even values and committed action. The therapist invited members to engage and participate while making it clear that they do not have to be feeling or thinking a certain way, which reflects getting present, willingness, defusion, self-as-context, and committed action. The therapist has already begun to embody key principles of the ACT model. She is modeling being present, defusion, and willingness in transparently sharing what is personally going on during the session (e.g., "I find that trying to inform people about ACT can be tricky"). This in and of itself is also a nice representation of values and committed action.

Summary

We began with a discussion of some of the challenges that come with applying ACT as a model and how to work with these in a useful way. We examined the overall trajectory of an ACT group, including the specific skills we are targeting in the therapy. We talked about the tools we use to develop these abilities and discussed ways to approach the therapy so that all the core processes are covered. We then moved to specific treatment planning and how an ACT therapist might approach an initial session. We discussed clinical decision making in ACT and provided some guidelines that can help the therapist remain within the model while moving things forward. Finally, we provided a sense of what an initial session might look like in the room. Let's move now to our first behavioral pillar, openness, and explore how to develop this in our group.

CHAPTER 5

Developing Willingness

Willingness, also referred to as *acceptance* in ACT, refers to the ability to experience one's thoughts, feelings, and bodily sensations without engaging in control or avoidance strategies, to "…have what's there to be had without needless defense" (Hayes et al., 2011, pp. 96–97). It represents an active choice, a stance one is choosing to take. It is a radical departure from how group members typically relate to their internal experiences, particularly those that are painful or uncomfortable in some way. We can see how this shift alters the function of such experiences. That is, they become something to notice, rather than something to fix or get out of.

As with the other core processes, willingness involves other abilities (contacting the present, self-as-context, values, and committed action), and these abilities also enable willingness. At this point in the therapy, our therapist wants to introduce the concept of willingness and help members begin to practice. She will be helping them develop willingness throughout the therapy, anticipating their abilities will build as she brings in the other processes.

This chapter picks up the group in session 1 after the therapist has completed introductions and the basic group tasks as described in chapter 4. We have discussed the challenge she faces immediately upon starting: she needs to create an opening for members to learn something new within a context that pulls for old, inflexible behavior (e.g., striving to control, avoid, or otherwise fix unwanted thoughts, feelings, and bodily sensations). Creating this opening will be the major thrust of this first session, but it is only a piece of the larger challenge. Ultimately she aims for her group members to learn to relate to their internal experiences in an entirely different way, and she intends to introduce willingness as part of that alternative in session 2.

Putting Willingness into Action

We join our therapist now as she walks her group through a process geared to evoke creative hopelessness ("hopeless" because efforts to control or avoid unwanted internal experiences don't ultimately work, and "creative" because recognizing this makes room for something new). Once the futility and cost of the control or fix-me agenda has been illuminated, the therapist will spend some time on the nature of misapplied control ("misapplied" because it is in the service of controlling what can't be controlled). She will then introduce the concept of willingness explicitly to the group by means of psychoeducation, group discussion, metaphors, and experiential exercises. Finally, we will observe how she goes about determining whether the group is ready to move to the next core process.

How to Evoke Creative Hopelessness

As our therapist demonstrates the process of evoking creative hopelessness, we will see how this procedure helps her meet the objectives she identified for her first session (described in the previous chapter). To recap, she will continue to develop a group culture that promotes psychological flexibility. She will also gain information she can use to develop an ACT conceptualization of her group members. Finally, she will be able to reveal the control or fix-me agenda as futile and costly, opening the way to an alternative approach. (Note that there is no need for the therapist to use clinical terms such as "creative hopelessness" or "psychological flexibility" with her group; we use them here for instructional purposes.)

Eliciting the Perceived Problem

It is time for our therapist to learn more about her group members, including what brings them to the group, what they perceive as the problem in their lives, and what they feel is needed. She will be looking through that ACT lens as she generates this discussion, assessing where their abilities lie in terms of the core processes and the degree to which a control or fix-it agenda might be functioning in unworkable ways.

Therapist: *(getting up and standing by the whiteboard)* Let's start by talking about why you are here. What isn't working in your lives? *(During this discussion, the therapist solicits participation as needed, simply listening if members are coming forward and participating, or eliciting participation by looking at various members invitingly or asking them direct questions.)*

Barry: *(after a pause)* Um, well, I'm just really depressed. I've got no friends…my family doesn't talk to me. *(The therapist quickly jots down "depression" on the whiteboard, and next to it draws an up arrow that signifies having too much depression. Then she writes "friends" with a down arrow [meaning not enough friends], and finally "family relationships" next to another down arrow. She then turns and looks inquiringly at the group.)*

Barry:	I haven't been doing well for a while. I lost my job about four months ago. I've gained thirty-two pounds in the last three months. I don't seem to care about anything anymore. (*Since "lost job" doesn't so easily lend itself to the arrow idea, the therapist just jots "lost job" on the board, then the word "weight" with an up arrow next to it, then "caring" with a down arrow.*)
Dan:	I have a job but I hate it! My ex-wife is trying to ruin my life…nothing is working out. (*Therapist writes down "job" and "ex-wife" and then "working out" with a down arrow.*)
Therapist:	What about you, Gina?
Gina:	I don't really know. My life has never worked.
Therapist:	What do you think is missing? (*Therapist decides to dig a bit deeper into this very general response. She ultimately wants to understand what Gina is and is not doing such that her life doesn't "work."*)
Gina:	I've never really accomplished anything. I don't have any motivation…also I don't have any friends, not really. My "friends" (*makes air quotes*) don't really care about me. (*Therapist writes "accomplishment," "motivation," and "caring friends" on the board, all with down arrows.*)
Therapist:	What is standing in the way of having more meaningful friendships?
Gina:	I don't know. I don't really trust people anyway; they always end up hurting you. (*Therapist writes "trust" on the board, with a down arrow beside it, then "hurt" with an up-arrow indicating too much hurt.*)

The therapist considered moving on to someone else after Gina made the comment about not having friends who really cared about her. She plans on learning more about what all her group members see as standing in their way very shortly. However, the global, external nature of Gina's comment (that none of her friends care about her) led our therapist to want to work with it a bit. Notice the therapist's precise use of language: "What is standing in the way of having more meaningful friendships?" Rather than align with Gina's categorization of her friends as being uncaring, the therapist subtly points to the qualities of the relationship between friends. This is more consistent with the model, placing "caring" as a behavior as opposed to a thing that is in a person or not. It also points to a domain (i.e., how people behave in a relationship) where Gina actually has some agency. Gina's response suggests fusion with rules (e.g., I can't trust, people always hurt you), and our therapist hypothesizes such rules are influencing Gina's behavior in ways that are problematic. We can imagine that as the therapy unfolds and Gina is brought into contact with her values, she could begin to build relationships that are personally meaningful. For now, the therapist takes in this information and files away her hypothesis—she will be keeping it in mind as she continues to move through the therapy.

The therapist continues with this exercise until the various concerns of the group are represented on the board. Now she wants to better understand the perceived barriers. Like Gina, members commonly provide external reasons for why their lives aren't working out (e.g., "my family," "my job"). While such situations are no doubt real stressors, they are not causal in the way that group members are thinking. How they are responding to these challenges could well be what is keeping them stuck. So while it is important to understand how group members perceive their situations, the therapist also wants to uncover how members respond to these situations and how that then functions in their lives.

Therapist: So what goes on for you with these things? (*to Dan*) How does the situation with your ex-wife stand in your way, for example?

Dan: I feel like she's turning my daughters against me. Seems like they'd rather be with her than me…we used to be close and now we hardly talk. (*Dan stops talking as he contacts his emotions.*)

Therapist: (*sits silently and compassionately for a bit in order to make room for the emotion that's shown up, modeling the core processes of contacting the present and willingness, then gently continues*) That sounds really painful. (*pausing again to sit with the feelings before continuing*) What's it like for you when you experience this, when you have those thoughts about your daughters not wanting to be with you?

Dan: I just feel like a loser! Unloved… (*pauses briefly*) I'm just so pissed that this has happened, that my wife just blew apart our family!

Keeping in mind that she can form only initial hypotheses at this point, our therapist noted that as Dan came into contact with the pain and vulnerability of feeling unloved, he quickly moved away into anger and into (again) how his wife is the problem. This reaction informs the therapist as to how Dan, at least in some situations, responds to uncomfortable thoughts and feelings. It suggests rigidity—Dan seems very caught up in this narrative about his family. She gets the sense he spends a lot of time (is highly fused) with these sorts of thoughts. As always, the therapist must make a clinical decision as to how best to respond to what has been shared. She could delve deeper into this issue with Dan, asking, for example, "How do you respond to those sorts of thoughts and feelings when they show up: being a 'loser,' or 'unloved'?"

This question is aimed at determining some of the specific strategies Dan employs and whether he finds these helpful and ultimately workable. She is wondering whether anger and blaming function to stave off more painful feelings. She could also ask, "Is that a new experience for you or have you felt that way before in your life?" This question assesses Dan's ability to observe his own experience (a core ACT process) and is a subtle intervention (Dan is invited to view his situation from another perspective, which could further learning to respond to it more flexibly). It also points to self-as-context, meaning the awareness that is constant through time and larger than the experiences of the moment.

The therapist could make a more general statement to the group: "I'm struck by the pain experienced in this group. Life can really be hard sometimes, can't it?" This group-level intervention could serve multiple functions. (Remember, though, that how an intervention actually functions is determined by the consequences that follow.) The therapist's observation demonstrates her awareness of the group's experience and could thus build rapport. Highlighting members' shared experience of pain could also build group cohesion and mutual compassion. While further demonstrating her compassion for the group, the second statement, "Life can be really hard…" is aimed at normalizing the experience of suffering, an ACT-consistent outcome. This very notion undermines the fix-it agenda; perhaps it's not that the group needs to get fixed so much as that pain is a part of the human experience.

In our hypothetical session, the discussion about barriers continues until all the members have participated. One thing the therapist is careful to avoid is getting caught up in the content. She gathers enough information to understand how group members perceive their situations (e.g., I lost my job, the problem is my ex-wife) but does not stay with content-level details (e.g., what happened at his job; what his ex-wife is or isn't doing). The key isn't even the internal experiences that members believe to be problematic (e.g., not having enough trust, motivation, or confidence, or having too much depression or anxiety), so much as how these experiences are functioning in the individual's life. What guides her clinical decision making here is remembering that the goal is to flush out the idea that "the problem" is having the wrong sort of internal experiences, and that these need to be fixed or replaced with better ones before one can live a good life. Any of the offered life issues could be further explored, analyzed, or problem solved, but the therapist seeks to highlight the common processes that help explain how her group members have become stuck.

In chapter 4 we discussed considerations that go into clinical decision making. Let's take another look at some of these in terms of what has occurred thus far in our hypothetical group:

Process over content: We have seen that the therapist is listening to the content of what group members are saying but also attending to the core processes potentially in play. She is considering how thoughts, feelings, and other behaviors function in members' lives, in the session, and in the moment at hand. When opportunities to build core processes arise, such as willingness to experience what's showing up in session, she takes them (e.g., modeling simply sitting with what's in the room).

Timing: As always, timing plays a significant role in what our therapist does in session. There is much she could say and do in response to what's being shared, but she is biding her time in order to make room for the information she is seeking. She is at the start of the therapy and has yet to explicitly discuss the core ACT processes. She is not expecting group members to demonstrate facility with them. If this discussion with Dan had arisen later in the therapy, the therapist might have invited the group to use it as an example of how to apply all the core processes (i.e., how Dan could work with the situation with his ex in a more value-driven way). For now, she simply makes a mental note of Dan's response while keeping the discussion at more of a group level.

Explicit versus nonexplicit intervention: Another consideration of our therapist is whether to use explicit or nonexplicit interventions. Because she is just getting started, she is working indirectly with much of what comes up in session, waiting until she has specifically introduced the core processes before calling them out explicitly. Using the dialogue with Dan as an example, the therapist has not yet introduced the concepts of getting present, defusion, self-as-process, or self-as-context, but she points to all these by asking questions such as "What's it like for you *when you experience* those sorts of thoughts?" Similarly, comments such as "It looks as though something powerful is *showing up for you* right now" and "Are you *having some of that experience* in this moment as we talk about this?" help her asses Dan's skill level with core ACT processes (e.g., defusion, self-as-context) while potentially helping him begin to build these abilities.

Experiential versus didactic work: This session would be very different if the therapist were relying upon didactic methods alone. We can imagine her trying to explain how efforts to control aren't workable and how willingness leads to more flexibility…and the subsequent positioning, defensiveness, or tuning out that could result. We can imagine a session that consists solely of an exchange of information, and how easy it would be for members to miss its import or dismiss it entirely. By eliciting the group members' own experiences and joining with them as they unfold in session, the therapist helps the group members experientially contact the struggle they've been in. She works to demonstrate that as a human being she has similar struggles. This reduces the need to defend and creates an opportunity to model how to simply sit with the pain of being human.

Illuminating the Futility of the Control or Fix-Me Agenda

At this point, the whiteboard is filled with up and down arrows next to a bunch of stated barriers. The therapist now wants to help the group contact the pain, futility, and cost of this control or fix-me agenda. (We like to use a dual-sided whiteboard for this next discussion so that we can continue to write down what is being generated while retaining what was previously recorded. Using sheets of butcher paper can create the same effect.)

Therapist: (*next to the blank whiteboard, prepared to write*) Let's take a different tack now. You've all shared some of the ways in which you are suffering, ways in which your lives aren't working out… I'm wondering how you've dealt with this stuff. What are some or the things you've tried?

Dan: I sleep a lot. And spend too much time on the computer. (*Therapist quickly jots "sleep" and "computer" on the board.*)

Brenda: I used to go running, but I don't even do that anymore. (*Therapists jots "go running" and "stop running" on the board.*)

Mary: Eating. I eat to numb-out a lot.

Therapist: (*writing "eating" and "numb-out" as she speaks; a quick pace helps get a lot of ideas flowing*) Yeah. How about chocolate? Anyone else use that? What about getting lost in a book or a movie? (*adds these to the board*)

The therapist's contribution here is consistent with the ACT model. She pointedly joins the group in its collective struggle, communicating that this is a human struggle and that she is in the same boat. Typically there is no shortage of control or fix-me strategies. The therapist can assist by asking whether members have tried to figure things out, turn over a new leaf, make a geographical move, and so on. (We like to encourage a lively discussion at the start of this exercise, but as the strategies pile up we allow ourselves to become more somber, contacting the pain of the struggle this represents. It is often the case—and fittingly so—that as the exercise continues, a heaviness enters the room.) Our therapist also becomes more somber as things progress, and she punctuates this by soliciting information regarding how many years group members have been struggling, how many medical providers they've seen, how many different treatments they've tried, and how many medications they have been on at one time or another. As is typical in a group setting, the aggregate number is quite large, and the group becomes still as she writes the totals on the board:

Therapist: (*circling the numbers as she speaks very seriously*) Hmmm. Looks like…thirty-five different doctors…around eighteen different treatments, forty-two meds… How many years are represented in this struggle (*adding*)…102? (*writes the number on the board and circles it*)

Let's pause again to talk about style. It is extremely important that the therapist be *in the experience* with the group. Conducting this exercise in a teachy, matter-of-fact way can easily be experienced as invalidating. Likewise, if the therapist is only focused on the points she is trying to make, she can miss what is actually happening in the room. It is critical that the suffering here be recognized, but in a way that does not support the very ideas and behaviors that have been keeping group members stuck. By being genuinely and compassionately interested in their experience, by being present to the group and whatever arises in the course of the discussion, the therapist builds a context wherein the group members feel understood. This in turn facilitates their ability to experience the bind they have been in non-defensively.

Now that the therapist has helped the group members experientially contact the struggle they are in, she is well-positioned to point even more clearly to the cost and futility of the control or fix-me agenda.

Therapist:	*(steps back from the board, thoughtfully looking it over for a bit)* I'm wondering what you all are making of this. What comes up for you when you look at all this?
	(Barry gives a big sigh.)
Therapist:	What are you experiencing, Barry?
Barry:	It's just…a lot of crap.
Mary:	Yeah, all that stuff…it's depressing. *(members nod in agreement)*
Therapist:	*(makes room for what's shown up in the room, just joining with the group in pondering the board for a while. As compassionately as possible, she eventually remarks)* Yeah. I'm feeling really moved by the struggle here. So many things you have tried! Moving, exercising, drinking, distracting, figuring it out, trying harder…forty-two medications! Years and years of struggle. *(pause)* Yes, I see a lot of suffering here. *(The group members silently assent, very in touch with their shared pain.)*
Therapist:	There's something else I'm seeing too. What strikes you about all this?
Barry:	*(after a pause)* It doesn't work. All that stuff… I'm still depressed.
Therapist:	*(leaning in)* Yes! All that effort and ingenuity…there's no lack of trying here. And yet…here you are. *(Group is silent.)*
Therapist:	I'm going to put out there that this stuff doesn't work because it doesn't work. *(Group regards her silently.)* All these ways to not have what you have? It doesn't work. *(leaning in)* Not for you, not for me, not for anybody. *(Therapist lets this sink in for a few moments. She flips the board, revealing the previously generated list of perceived barriers with their up or down arrows.)* You have been striving to have less of this *(pointing to "depression")* or this *(pointing to anxiety)*. Or working to have more of this *(pointing to "confidence")* or waiting to have more of this *(pointing to "motivation")*.

You have worked hard! And yet, from what you have shared today, it seems that it has not worked. And I want to put out there that this is not about you. This isn't some failure in you, something you just have to work harder at or just figure out so you can finally pull it off. We already have that up there (*indicating "work harder" and "figure it out" on the board*). You've tried that already. And yet, here you are. (*Therapist pauses, then continues very clearly and very compassionately.*) This agenda, to be more, better, or different, to be fixed so that we don't have what we have, isn't doable. It is a hopeless agenda. (*Therapist lets this sink in and just sits with the group as they digest what she has said. She eventually continues*):

Maybe you've been thinking this is something about you—that something is wrong with you because you haven't been able to pull this off. This is a *human nature* problem. Somewhere we get the idea that we shouldn't be experiencing what we're experiencing and then we try to get rid of it. Or we wait until we feel a certain way before we live the way we want to be living. But check your own experience—how well has that worked?

Our therapist has now poked a hole in the idea that if group members could just get fixed, unwanted internal experiences would be gone from their lives. Her group is beginning to comprehend that this therapy is not going to be in pursuit of that agenda. The result is often confusion, fear, anger…sometimes even relief as members connect with their own experiential knowledge that what they've been unsuccessfully striving for is unattainable (and maybe it's not about them!). The ways in which individual members react to this provides a demonstration of the very topic being discussed.

Mary:	(*looking anxious and a bit frustrated*) So are you saying that there's nothing that can be done?
Therapist:	I'm asking what your own experience with this has been. What have you discovered?
Mary:	So what's the answer then?
Therapist:	Do you mind if I point something out right now? (*Mary somewhat grudgingly shakes her head.*) Right now it looks as though you are experiencing something uncomfortable. What are you feeling?
Mary:	I don't know what you're getting at here. You're saying nothing works.
Therapist:	(*resisting the urge to point out it is Mary's experience that is saying nothing works*) What are you feeling right now? What emotions?

Mary:	I'm frustrated!
Therapist:	Yeah. And is there some fear there?
Mary:	(*suddenly not looking angry but vulnerable*) Yeah.
Therapist:	Yeah. And it seems that one way of dealing with that is to ask questions, to figure it out. (*Mary hesitates, nods. The therapist adds "ask questions" and "figure it out" on the board.*)

We must again stress the importance of therapist style. Real skill is required here. The therapist is boldly challenging the unworkable control or fix-me agenda while also working to convey compassion for the pain of this very human dilemma: not wanting to experience pain while not being able to avoid pain, and then having the pain of that very struggle on top of everything else. Verbal and nonverbal behaviors (e.g., facial expression, posture, pace, tone) that convey understanding and kindness are crucial here.

Imagine now that after a short pause, Dan bursts out with "This is bullshit!" Imagine next that the therapist simply nods very understandingly, then writes, "get angry" on the board, and waits interestedly for the next response. This is an example of how liberating being facile with ACT can be—an experience eventually reported by nearly everyone we have trained or supervised in the therapy. That is, in accordance with the model, the therapist does not have to come up with a solution to Dan's anger. What is happening in this moment is not a "problem" per se. In recognizing how this behavioral response functions, the therapist is guided to respond in a way that furthers the therapy. Notice how this does not mean she ignores Dan's anger or invalidates him in some way. With facial expression and attitude she treats his anger as important while raising the possibility that this could actually be a way for Dan to deal with other, more difficult feelings.

This is also where group work really adds to the therapeutic power of ACT. That is, even if in the moment Dan is unable to consider whether getting angry is a way for him to handle discomfort, it is quite possible that other members of the group will understand and learn from the interaction. The opportunity to observe how behavioral processes manifest in others greatly enables members to see these same processes in their own behavior.

It is helpful to remember the overarching objective of this session. Therapists can feel very pulled in such moments to fix what is happening in the room (e.g., to alleviate fears, soothe uncertainty, resolve confusion). Such a response by the therapist would actually demonstrate the very behavior being stressed as problematic. It can also be helpful to remember that she is not needing group members to suddenly shift to another way of approaching things; that is where she hopes to ultimately land in ACT. At this point, she is simply pointing to the elephant in the room—the notion that efforts to have different thoughts, feelings, and sensations don't actually work—and highlighting the pain of being in that struggle.

Dan: So if there's no point, then why are we here?

Therapist: (*pausing to fully consider her thoughts*) I need to be careful here, because I find myself wanting to reassure you and give you answers as a way to feel more comfortable. It's hard to sit with my own anxiety about what you all are experiencing right now. But that would be more of the same, wouldn't it? (*goes to the board and writes "provide answers" on the list of strategies*) I think I do want to say that yes, there is a point to what we are doing here. There is a direction we are headed. For now, though, I simply point to the terrible struggle you've been in. I'm wondering if we can just be in touch with that right now.

When more dialogue seems problematic, turning to an experiential exercise or metaphor can be a good move. Doing so here not only helps the therapist make her point about the futility of the control agenda, but also helps her refrain from aligning with attempts to alleviate discomfort. The therapist accordingly pulls in the man-in-a-hole metaphor to illustrate the futility of the control or fix-me agenda.

Therapist: I'm going to use a metaphor to help describe what we're talking about here. Imagine that you have been blindfolded and that you cannot take this blindfold off. And imagine that you have been dropped into a field and told, "Go live your life." So you march off, but unbeknownst to you, that field is full of holes. (*pauses*) What do you think will eventually happen, if you're wandering around blindfolded in a field full of holes?

Mary: You're going to fall in!

Therapist: You're going to fall in. But being human, you want out of there, so you feel around and find a tool, just one tool. You find a shovel. (*pauses*) So you start digging. And digging. (*pauses again*) But what happens when you're in a hole and you're digging?

Dan: You dig yourself in deeper.

Therapist: (*simply sits for a moment or two, letting this sink in*) The hole gets deeper. (*sits*)

Therapist: (*eventually continuing, indicating the list of strategies on the board*) You've been in a hole, and you've been digging. (*pauses*) And, anything I offer to you right now? You would probably dig with it. (*sits with the group as they ponder this silently*) So right now, I simply invite you to see that you've been digging.

At this point our therapist determines she has accomplished her goals for session 1. She has started off the group, completed basic tasks, and begun to create a therapeutic environment that is

ACT-consistent. She has gathered information on where members stand in terms of psychological flexibility and developed hypotheses as to why they have been stuck. She has pulled out the problematic control or fix–me agenda that would stand in the way of therapy if left unaddressed. She believes she helped the group contact the futility and cost of this agenda (i.e., creative hopelessness) and managed to refrain from attempting to fix or soften this awareness.

The main reason the therapist believes she has been successful in evoking creative hopelessness is the reaction of her group members. That is, members appear nonplussed, confused, a bit afraid, and not a little curious. Given the implications of what they have covered in the session—that this group is not going to be about pursuing a control or fix-me agenda (the very thing they had hoped to receive)—a blithe "Okay, what's next?" reaction would be suspect. As she observes these varying responses, our therapist seizes the opportunity to help her group begin to work with such experiences in a different way. She sits in silence, allowing herself to fully experience what's in the room (and modeling this for the group) and elects to end the session simply, careful not to take away from the moment by suddenly changing tone.

Therapist: I think we've done our work for today. I will see you all next Tuesday.

Session Strategy. At this point in the therapy, the therapist has pointed to the futility of the fix-me agenda and hopefully created an opening for something new. To further pave the way for willingness, she plans to spend the next session exploring the nature of misapplied control. Specifically, in session 2, our therapist plans to generate a group discussion that covers the following points:

- Attempting to control unwanted internal events (thoughts, feelings, sensations) does not ultimately work.

- Efforts to control can have a paradoxical effect.

- Continuing to engage in this battle is quite costly.

Next, the therapist wants to move explicitly into willingness. She plans to provide psychoeducation regarding what is meant by willingness in ACT and to conduct experiential exercises that demonstrate the process and provide the group with opportunities for practice. She has several such exercises in mind and will allow herself to choose which ones (and how many) as the session unfolds.

Welcoming the group back for the second session, the therapist sets off with her plan in mind, knowing full well that her agenda may shift as the session unfolds.

The Problem with Misapplied Control

The therapist is mindful of the fact that group members have had a week between sessions and that it is likely much of what was accomplished in the first session has dimmed in their minds. For this reason she puts the list of unworkable strategies generated in the previous session back on the whiteboard where it can be seen by the group. (We either keep the original list on the whiteboard intact and use it again in this session or write the list on butcher paper so we can post it in future sessions.) Her first move is to revisit previous terrain:

Therapist:	So last week we came up with a lot of things we've tried in order to not have what we have (*gesturing to her chest to indicate internal phenomena*). I'm wondering what sorts of thoughts and feelings have shown up for you around last week's session.
Barry:	I tried not to think about it, to be honest.
Therapist:	(*interested, nodding understandingly*) Yeah (*looking over the list of strategies*). I think we have that one, don't we? Yes, here it is: don't think about it. (*underlines it*)
Gina:	I don't even remember what we talked about last week! (*The therapist adds "forget" to the board, then waits for other responses by group members. This doesn't mean she won't provide a recap—in fact she does so shortly. For now, though, this response keeps the therapist on track with learning where the group is as a whole. Adding this to the list also subtly raises the question as to how "forgetting" might be functioning for Gina.*)
Therapist:	(*after the group members have had a chance to share their various thoughts and feelings*) And then we arrived at kind of a tough place, didn't we? We landed on how all these strategies ultimately don't work. (*pauses and just sits with the group, reflecting for a bit*) That's where I'd like to go today: What if the larger problem here is all that trying? What if control itself is more the culprit here?

At this point the therapist has reoriented the group, reestablishing the bind that is created by pursuing the control or fix-me agenda. She has explicitly pointed to control as the culprit and is well placed to begin exploring it further.

Now that the problematic control agenda is on the table, our therapist wants to examine it more fully with her group. Her hope is that members will become increasingly clear on the futility and cost of this agenda in order to further pave the way for willingness. The following simple exercises point to the futility of this sort of control.

What Are the Numbers?
(futility of misapplied control)

(Hayes et al., 2011)

This simple exercise neatly points out the inherent difficulty in trying not to think a particular thought. The therapist picks three numbers (we typically make it simple: "Let's say the numbers are one, two, and three") and makes sure the group is clear on what they are. She then instructs the group that for the next minute or so, their task is to *not* think about those numbers. The response is nearly always a quick realization that this task is not possible. Even if a group member were to report, "I did it!" the therapist could quickly point out the paradox here: "How do you know you did it? Because you weren't thinking about…what?" (In other words, the referent must be present in order to know one is not thinking about it.)

Next, the therapist conducts another exercise to further bring to light the futility of misapplied control. This exercise, called "Fall in Love," can be found in the Supplemental Exercises at http://www.newharbinger.com/23994.

These two exercises focus on the ineffectiveness of trying to control thoughts and feelings. The next exercise uses a metaphorical anxiety machine to demonstrate the futility of trying to control the physical sensations of anxiety (and anxious thoughts and feelings as well). It also demonstrates the paradoxical nature of control—that the harder one tries not to have a thought, a feeling, or a sensation, the more present it is. When conducting it in a group setting, it is important to speak to the group when possible and to solicit participation from everyone as the exercise unfolds.

Anxiety Machine Metaphor

(Hayes et al., 1999; Walser & Westrup, 2007; paradoxical effects of misapplied control)

Our therapist begins by asking for a volunteer (Mary volunteers). She then pretends to hook Mary up to an "exquisitely sensitive anxiety machine." The group is told that the machine is geared to register even the tiniest blip of anxiety. The therapist then earnestly informs Mary, "Your only job is to not feel anxious. Everything else is okay; just absolutely don't have any anxiety." As expected, Mary and the rest of the group are quick to see that the result of this instruction is an increase in anxiety. The therapist playfully responds by asking Mary to try harder, which of course only increases her anxiety. When she feels the point has been made, she takes a more somber tone and asks the group to notice that even in this playful, innocuous exercise it was impossible to make anxiety go away. She asks them to consider that in their actual lives the stakes are actually *much* higher, perhaps to the point of thinking, "I can't *live* unless my anxiety (or sadness, or insecurity, or anger) goes away."

Introducing Willingness as an Alternative

Once the group is in touch with the no-win battle against unwanted internal experiences, members are in a position to consider an alternative approach. Notice the use of the word "consider." That is, the therapist is not expecting her group members to suddenly stop engaging in control or avoidance strategies and move into acceptance of unwanted thoughts and feelings. Rather, her hope at this point is that they are at least considering willingness as an alternative. Here are the key points she wishes to make as they work with this core process:

- Willingness is *an alternative way* (not the "right" way) to respond to what members internally experience as they live their lives.

- Willingness is a stance, not a feeling.

- Willingness is not a concession.

- Willingness is an ability that can be developed.

Again, relying on teaching or persuading is unlikely to be effective here. Fortunately, there are many wonderful metaphors and exercises in the ACT literature that can be used to introduce willingness in an accessible way. In fact, we typically prefer to start experientially with the Tug-of-War exercise, described below. This exercise provides a segue from misapplied control as the problem to willingness, as it demonstrates both ideas nicely. It also works particularly well in a group setting, involving everyone and providing an opportunity for experiential learning.

Tug-of-War
(willingness as an alternative)

Our therapist has anticipated doing this exercise and has brought a rope with her to the session. (In lieu of a rope we have used belts and sweaters.)

Therapist: (*picking up the rope and standing before the group*) Okay, I need a volunteer! (*After some laughter and joking by the group about what the rope is for, Barry agrees to volunteer.*)

Therapist: Thank you Barry. (*Hands him one end of the rope*). What we're going to do is play tug-of-war (*she moves a distance away from Barry so they are in position where the group can comfortably observe them*). Most of you are familiar with how to play tug-of-war? (*Members nod*). So you are over there (*speaking to Barry*), I'm here, and between us is a deep chasm…an endless chasm. (*Barry nods.*) I am going to be what you are struggling with. What are you most struggling with at this point in your life?

Barry: Depression.

Therapist: (*nodding compassionately*) And what is it about depression that you find difficult? What do you find painful about that experience? [*Notice how the therapist is using language aimed at undermining depression as a "thing" that is in Barry or that somehow has landed on him. She is subtly guiding him to a more fine-grained observation of his experience with depression. This furthers his ability to observe self-as-process and also facilitates defusion and self-as-context, abilities that will be more fully explored in chapters 6 and 8.*]

Barry: (*getting more serious as he gets in contact with what he is saying*) I'm…just really lonely. It's lonely.

Therapist: (*verbal and nonverbal behavior appropriately tuned with what Barry is contacting*) Yes, loneliness is a pretty painful experience. (*pauses for a bit before continuing*) In this exercise I am going to represent your loneliness (*moves far enough away from Barry so that the rope is taut*). So I am that painful loneliness you have been struggling with. (*gives the rope a slight tug*)

Barry: (*pulling back slightly in response*) Okay.

Therapist: (*pulling a bit harder, tugging back and forth as Barry responds by doing the same*) And this is what we've been doing for…how long now?

Barry: (*looking a little tense*) What?

Therapist: How long have you been trying to deal with being lonely?

Barry: Oh. A long time.

Therapist: Years? (*Barry nods*) Do you remember when you first had the experience of being lonely? (*Note the word choice: "...had the experience."*)

Barry: (*growing somber*) Well...yeah, way back. (*Therapist waits, keeping the rope taught and giving a tug now and then.*) I remember feeling that way when I was eight or so.

Therapist: (*nods very compassionately, clearly moved by what Barry is saying*) Eight years old... that's a long time!

Barry: (*looking sad now*) Yeah.

Therapist: And so I've been in your life for years now...and you've been struggling with me. You've tried all sorts of things in fact (*therapist nods her head at the ever-present list of control or fix-me strategies*). But I'm still here (*pulling harder*).

Barry: (*pulling back harder in response*) Yeah.

Therapist: (*after a bit, continuing to pull*) So here we are.

Barry: (*looking sad*) Yeah.

Therapist: (*to the group*) So, this doesn't seem to be working. This constant tugging, pulling, working to have me be gone. Barry's been at this for years now (*nodding her head toward the ever-present list of strategies*). As we've seen, we can all spend years here. (*pauses to let this sink in while continuing to tug on the rope*) So it looks like we're in agreement that this doesn't work too well. Any ideas what else might be done?

Barry: I can just ignore you.

Therapist: (*gives a sharp tug on the rope, Barry tugs back reflexively*) Have you tried that? Ignoring your loneliness?

Barry: Yeah... (*Therapist says nothing, but continues to keep the rope taut.*)

Mary: (*chiming in*) Drop the rope!

Gina: Go over to her side! (*Barry looks questioningly at the therapist, who gives a tug and gazes back impassively.*)

Barry: (*nodding at the "chasm" between them*) So what, I just give in?

Therapist: What would "giving in" do?

Barry: Well, maybe you'd stop bugging me.

Therapist:	So you give in to loneliness so that it doesn't bother you as much?
Barry:	Yeah!
Therapist:	(*addressing the group while still tugging on the rope*) Could someone please add that to our list? Giving in?
Barry:	(*comprehending*) Oh.
Therapist:	Yeah. That would be another tug wouldn't it? Giving in so that I get smaller or go away is just another way to be in this battle with me.
Several group members:	Drop the rope! (*Barry hesitantly drops the rope. The therapist picks it up and hands it back to him without saying anything, and he takes it back. The therapist tugs and Barry tugs back.*)
Barry:	Okay…
Therapist:	Yeah, here we are again…
Dan:	Just drop the rope! (*Barry looks inquiringly at the therapist, who simply gazes back, then he hesitantly drops the rope. The therapist picks it up and starts to hand it to him.*)
Mary:	Don't take it! Don't take it back! (*Barry hesitates but refuses to take the rope.*)
Therapist:	Wait, are you sure you don't want to take this? (*Barry shakes his head.*) But, I need you to struggle with me! Don't you want to pull some more? (*More sure, Barry shakes his head.*)
Barry:	Nope!
	(*The therapist assesses the group, checking to see where members are at. Members are nodding and smiling, indicating they are with Barry on this.*)
Therapist:	So this is interesting. You have dropped the rope—what is that like for you?
Barry:	It feels better… I'm not pulling so hard. Like I'm free.
Therapist:	(*to the group, with emphasis*) Yeah, you're not in that ongoing, exhausting battle. But notice something here (*raising her voice and calling out to Barry*): I'm still heeeerrreee! I'm your loneliness and I'm still here! (*pauses while the group thinks this over*)
Barry:	Yeah, but I'm not fighting with you. You're just there.

Therapist: Yes! And notice this: just walk around the room a bit. (*As Barry moves around the room, the therapist follows.*) I'm still here, but you're no longer stuck in this struggle. (*Therapist mimes being fully engaged in an intense tug-of-war, feet planted, eyes locked on an imagined adversary.*) You are free to go where you choose to go, *if* you are willing to drop the rope. And I'll still be here…(*raising her voice*) sometimes really loud, (*more softly*) sometimes just hanging around in the background. (*Therapist sees that Barry is looking downcast.*) What's happening for you Barry?

Barry: (*sighing heavily*) I wish… I just wish I didn't have this.

Therapist: (*very compassionately*) Yeah. (*pausing for a bit*) And how often have you had that thought?

Barry: A lot.

Therapist: Yeah. (*very gently*) We should probably add that to our list: "wishing it away." I know I've had that thought, has anyone else? (*Every group member assents.*)

Barry: But that just keeps me stuck with it.

Therapist: Yes. (*to the group, leaning in*) Trying not to have this stuff keeps us in this battle that can't be won. This therapy is about the *rope* (*pointing to the rope*). It's about the struggle with difficult thoughts and feelings, and the cost of that struggle (*again miming being in a tug-of-war while continuing*). Here we are, engaged in this struggle for years and years, while meanwhile, what's not happening?

Mary: We're not going anywhere.

Therapist: (*with a sweeping gesture to indicate the room and beyond*) Life is passing us by!

At this point the therapist feels the group has received what she intended with this exercise. She thanks Barry and asks him to rejoin the circle to continue the discussion. Now that the group has some understanding of what is meant by willingness in ACT, she can discuss it more fully.

We will comment here that we love to use this exercise in group settings because it is so active and easily engages everyone. In fact, a protracted, even emotionally painful struggle between the therapist and volunteer only makes the point more strongly.

We have also found that the concept of willingness, as meant in ACT, is often misunderstood. It will be important for our therapist to spend some time assessing how her group members are hearing what she is saying. In particular, we have found it essential to make the following two points:

- *Willingness is not a feeling.* It is important for the therapist to clarify that willingness is not about the feeling of wanting. As it applies to Barry, this isn't about him wanting his loneliness, or otherwise feeling differently about it. Rather, this is about being willing to have the experience of loneliness, which would include his own reactions to that (e.g., not wanting it). The therapist can help Barry and the others understand that this is about the struggle itself—the rope—not what's on the other side of the chasm.

- **Willingness is not a concession.** Along with helping her group members grasp that willingness is a stance and not a feeling, the therapist will need to help them differentiate willingness from concession or resignation. Far from giving in or giving up, choosing to "drop the rope" is an intentional, powerful move. It is choosing to no longer engage in an unwinnable battle in order to get on with the business of living.

To help make this point, the therapist asks Barry how he felt when he realized he didn't actually have to pick up the rope, even when "loneliness" was telling him that he must. Not surprisingly, Barry reports he felt empowered, adding "but it was hard to know it was still there." This last comment indicates Barry understands how willingness is conceived in ACT. Being willing does not make unwanted experiences go away, but letting go of the struggle increases flexibility.

Let's check back in with our therapist. At this point, willingness has been introduced, and from what she has gleaned from their participation, members are understanding what this process is about. Bear in mind that she has been looking for ways to actively engage the group in willingness as a choice throughout the session. She has utilized in-the-moment opportunities whenever possible, asking, for example, "Did you notice how quickly we moved off that topic a moment ago? I'm wondering if you would be willing to just sit with me for a moment, noticing what's coming up for us around this."

If time allowed, our therapist could conduct another willingness exercise. However, as she assesses her group, it seems the Tug-of-War exercise truly resonated and that anything more might take away from that experience. She is also considering the next session and knows that the next core process to tackle is defusion; however, she is aware that willingness is not an easy ability to master. (Do we ever?) She decides to hold off for now, thinking it might work well to begin the next session with the Eyes On exercise (Hayes et al., 1999) to provide an additional in-the-moment opportunity to practice willingness.

To close today's session, the therapist asks the group members to tune in to what they are experiencing in the moment. She asks them to notice the thoughts showing up, the emotions, and any physical sensations. She models contacting the present in this way by sitting quietly with them for a few moments, noticing her own experience. After a bit, she remarks on the fact that regardless of what is showing up, they all seem able to simply notice and hold their experience—to choose to be willing. She invites them to experiment with this as they go about their lives during the next week, and then ends the session.

Clinical Considerations in Working with Willingness

Process versus content: The "creative hopelessness" procedure is designed to highlight process rather than content. That is, when generating a list of all the things the group members have tried to fix their internal experiences, the focus is not so much on the strategies themselves (their content or form) but on how they function. What are they in the service of? Do they work? What are the consequences? A particular strategy might be "good" at a content or form level (e.g., exercise), but if it is functioning in a problematic way (e.g., the group member is striving to use exercise as way to escape marital tension), it is worth looking at. Rather than fall into the trap of persuasion or cajoling, we guide the group members to their own recognition of how efforts to control function in their lives.

Timing: While there are innumerable ways to introduce and work with the core processes in ACT, we like to start with willingness as a way to put the problematic fix-it agenda "on notice." We anticipate the control agenda will appear regularly throughout the therapy, and we find that putting it on the table at the outset as problematic helps the group recognize it when it occurs.

Explicit versus nonexplicit intervention: In this section we saw how the therapist began with *doing* over explaining. She modeled sitting with what was unfolding in the session and worked with members in a way that provided opportunities for them to do the same (i.e., retraining from answering questions that are attempts to get out of discomfort). By ending the first session with the man-in-a-hole metaphor, the group members were faced with just sitting with their reactions to being stuck. By providing these types of instances of experiencing paving the way, we become well placed to explicitly name willingness as a targeted ability in ACT. We are able to point to earlier instances as examples, and once willingness has been specifically explored as a group, we continue to highlight opportunities as they unfold.

Experiential versus didactic learning: The therapist has drawn heavily upon experiential learning to introduce and begin to develop willingness in her group members. She evoked a situation (creative helplessness) to help the group contact the pain of an unworkable control or fix-it agenda. Likewise, she utilized experiential exercises that were far more effective than didactic explanations. Just consider the difference in impact between offering statements such as "If you try not to have a thought, you have the thought" and tasking the group to actually try not to think about certain numbers. The simple exercises described in this section not only are effective teaching tools, but also add liveliness and spark to the session.

Summary

In this chapter our therapist began the core work of ACT. After having completed the basic tasks and set an ACT-consistent tone for the therapy, she took the group through the process of creative hopelessness, managing to pull out the problematic control agenda and highlighting its unworkability. Relying primarily on experiential exercises, she helped the group understand the problems with misapplied control and introduced willingness as an alternative.

While these ideas certainly pave the way for being open to experience, doing so as life unfolds takes a great deal of skill. Our minds have much to say about what is and is not okay, what we can and cannot tolerate. This is why being open in ACT involves not just willingness but the ability to relate to our thoughts in a way that reduces their influence. In the next chapter we will address how these important abilities are fostered in ACT.

CHAPTER 6

Building Defusion

In chapter 1 we examined the nature of thinking and how we "fall into" our thoughts, and then live in that verbal virtual reality to the point where it overshadows all else. In ACT we aim to help clients see thoughts for what they are so that they are freed to make choices according to their values. An inherent challenge is that the central feature of being fused with thoughts is an inability to see that one is fused! This is where group work can really help. Members are able to observe their peers' relationships with thoughts, which helps them see how they relate to their own.

In this chapter our therapist will guide her group to this very different way of relating to thoughts. Over the course of two sessions, we will see how she introduces the concept of *defusion* and then how she helps the group build their defusion skills. We will begin as she develops a plan for the group's third ACT session. An important part of her plan is to assess her group's progress thus far, and, as we saw in the last chapter, she has decided to spend some more time working on willingness before moving ahead. We will follow her as she conducts an experiential willingness exercise.

Next, we will see how our therapist introduces defusion to the group and goes about making sure members take away the points she considers central to developing this skill. Specifically, we will see how she uses psychoeducation, group discussion, metaphors, and experiential exercises to further the work, and we will join her in some of the clinical decision making that ensues. We will observe how she pulls in the topic of language itself as a means to help group members see thoughts as something they produce (rather than as literal truth). We conclude the chapter at the end of session 4 as the therapist assesses her group's progress and determines where to head next.

Putting Defusion into Action

In the first two sessions the therapist and her group worked on willingness. Her sense at the end of session 2 was that the group had received the main points she had wanted to get across. However, she knows that understanding and doing are very different things. Her experience also tells her that clients will often turn willingness into another strategy, along the lines of, *I'll just accept this so that then it will go away* (*be less bothersome*). She is therefore confident in her decision to do more work with willingness in session 3, emphasizing opportunities to practice, before beginning to work on building defusion.

> **Session Strategy.** As we followed our therapist through her decision-making process at the end of session 2, we learned that she plans to begin this session with the Eyes On exercise to reinforce the concept of willingness. She will also keep an eye out for willingness opportunities that arise during the session. She will spend the rest of the available time, and at least the following session, working on defusion. It can be a challenging skill to acquire, and she has found that a full session is generally needed to do justice to the role of language in thinking (and suffering). In this session, she intends to introduce defusion and help members learn to observe their thoughts. She will provide initial psychoeducation about what is meant by "looking at, versus from, thoughts" and will then conduct one or two exercises that will help illuminate this concept. As homework, she plans to ask her group members to notice any thoughts that keep them rigidly stuck in problematic patterns of behavior, and also that this entails looking *at* them instead of *from* them.

The therapist begins session 3 by welcoming members and conducting a brief mindfulness exercise. She then generates a discussion about what they have covered in the group so far, which both orients the group and provides her with important feedback. For example, she might ascertain from members' various reactions the degree to which they understand (or misconstrue) willingness, whether they remain invested in a control or fix-me agenda, or whether they see willingness as such a strategy. She is careful to engage everyone and to solicit information that will guide her decision making.

Moving from Willingness to Defusion

At the end of this discussion, our therapist has concluded that while some members seem to have a better grasp than others, overall the group shows a reasonable understanding of both the unworkability of misapplied control and what is meant by willingness as an alternative. She decides it is good timing to move from verbal to experiential learning, and she prepares to move into the Eyes On exercise (see the Supplemental Exercises at http://www.newharbinger.com/23994), which involves breaking members into pairs and having the partners sit closely across from one another, simply gazing without speaking. During the exercise, she is most interested to see whether or not members will engage in the exercise. The willingness opportunity is that members can choose to participate despite whatever comes up for them. Giggling, struggling, looking away then looking back—all are reactions to be noticed as opposed to signs of doing the exercise "wrong." After concluding the exercise, in fact, the therapist points out that those who struggled in this way and yet continued with the exercise demonstrated willingness quite nicely.

In processing the exercise with the group afterwards, the therapist is assessing the degree to which individual members are on board. For example, she might find that one or two members are still firmly invested in control as a strategy based on their comments following the exercise. In such a scenario, it might be prudent to revisit creative hopelessness and control as being the larger problem. However, in this instance, our therapist observed that all of her group members successfully participated in the exercise, continuing to engage with their partners despite their discomfort. Their comments during the group discussion following the exercise also led her to believe that members are starting to understand and experience what is meant by willingness in ACT. She determines they are ready to move ahead.

Introducing and Developing Defusion

In considering the core ACT process of defusion, the therapist's main goal is to help her group members learn how to relate to their thoughts in a way that leads to more flexible behavior. Specifically, she wants to help group members (1) learn to observe their thoughts, (2) learn to de-literalize their thoughts, and (3) increase their awareness of the distinction between Thinker and thought. Let's look at these a little more closely:

1. Observing thoughts: Being able to defuse from thoughts begins with the ability to look *at*, rather than *from*, thoughts. In other words, noticing a thought as a thought requires some ability to step out of it for a moment. The therapist will model this ability as much as possible throughout the session and will help group members begin to notice and talk about the thoughts they are experiencing. Employing mindfulness exercises in session (which includes bringing awareness to one's thoughts) and having members practice between sessions will also be key.

2. De-literalizing thoughts: The therapist wants her group to learn the difference between having a thought and "buying" a thought (meaning relating to it as being literally true). In pursuit of that goal, the therapist will demonstrate the powerful role language plays when it comes to thoughts and human suffering. She will seek to demonstrate how even very painful thoughts are the product of language and how we then come to relate to our thoughts in unworkable ways.

3. Distinguishing between Thinker and thoughts: As her group members begin to learn how to notice their thoughts and relate to them as a process to experience, the therapist will verbally direct their attention to the distinction between Thinker and thought. This points to experiencing self-as-context, though the therapist plans to explore that process explicitly later in the therapy. At this point she intends to simply bring attention to this distinction as a way to foster defusion.

Developing the Ability to Observe Thoughts

The therapist introduces this topic in a straightforward way: "Let's talk about the nature of thinking itself. Does anyone here know the difference between looking *at* rather than *from* thoughts?" She then provides some examples of the distinction ("Listen to the difference between *I'm such a loser* and *I'm having the thought that I'm a loser*") and discusses these differences with the group, highlighting the point that the latter seems to carry less meaning. Once they have a sense of this distinction, she moves into the Leaves on a Stream exercise (Hayes, 2005; available in the Supplemental Exercises at http://www.newharbinger.com/23994) to provide an experiential learning opportunity. She primes the group for what this particular exercise is targeting by stating it will provide them an opportunity to practice looking at, rather than from, thoughts.

After completing the exercise, the therapist allows plenty of time to process it with the group. She seeks opportunities to model, commenting, for example, "I noticed at one point that I'd gone completely downstream with a thought." She also works to remain focused on the targeted process rather than getting pulled into content.

Therapist:	I'd like to hear what you all experienced during that exercise.
Gary:	I couldn't do it.
Therapist:	Is that something you were thinking during the exercise? (*Gary nods.*) So, that thought, *I can't do this*, showed up at some point… Were you able to notice it and put it on a leaf, or did you go downstream with it a bit?

Or another process-oriented response:

Therapist:	So just now, you had the thought, *I can't do this*, is that right? (*Gary nods.*) Great, okay. Now let's see what the next thought is. (*waits with group members*)

The ACT literature is full of wonderful exercises that develop defusion in different ways. The Leaves on a Stream exercise focuses on the ability to notice the thought process itself. That is, group members are tasked with being able to observe their thought processes enough to capture and articulate thoughts as they arise. Viewing thoughts in this way is quite a shift, and our therapist wants to capitalize on that. Her next exercise, Silly Voices (Hayes, Pankey, Gifford, Batten, & Quiñones, 2002), targets the way in which distressing thoughts function for her group members. The ability to notice thoughts is furthered, as group members gain increased awareness of just how these particular ones have been functioning, and that in the end, they are just thoughts.

Silly Voices
(defusion)

The therapist reminds the group about discussions around languaging and defusion. She spends some time on this to ensure they have a good grasp on it. She then asks the group to think about a particular thought about themselves that is really painful, one that visits them frequently, such as things related to being "fat," "lazy," "stupid," or "inadequate." She instructs them to write a narrative—as if they were writing a journal entry—about that notion, including how it impacts them behaviorally and emotionally. She lets them know that these will be shared with the group and allows about five minutes for the writing task.

Next, the therapist asks everyone to go around the circle sharing what they wrote. She makes sure that no one "rescues" others from their thoughts, as doing so only lends credence to buying in to the thoughts. She has all the group members read their narratives in turn with no talking in between. She invites the group to notice how the room feels. Common descriptions are "heavy," "sad," and "connected."

She then instructs everyone to read exactly the same passage, but this time to do so in a silly voice. She allows them to be as creative as they can be, but for those who can't think of a voice, she suggests they plug their nose or stick their thumb in their mouth.

Last, the therapist leads a discussion about how the room feels now and why (pointing to the change in function of the identified thoughts), and what the personal experiences were for each group member. Checking in with the group after this exercise can be powerful, and it is unlikely that any of the group members have experienced treating their painful thoughts in such a light-hearted manner.

Session 3 is drawing to a close, and the therapist concludes the discussion. To help group members develop their skills outside of group, she asks them to continue to work on defusion for homework as they go about their lives. Specifically, she invites them to notice and check in with their thoughts from time to time "as though you're standing on the riverbank." She is careful to add that as they attempt this, their minds might hand them all sorts of evaluations about the exercise or how they're doing and that these are simply more thoughts to be noticed.

Now that her group members are learning to observe and relate differently to their thoughts, our therapist would like to spend the next session strengthening these skills. As we know, this is not an easy task. Let's learn how she goes about this work as she prepares for session 4.

Session Strategy. At the start of session 4, the therapist will follow up on her invitation to her group members to notice thoughts during the past week and will provide more psychoeducation if called for. She then plans to focus on the difference between noticing and buying thoughts, and again she has an exercise or two in mind to help her convey this distinction. She will specifically discuss the role of language, as she believes this piece will help group members come to relate to their thoughts as a behavior, something they are doing (which will help them take them less literally).

As usual, the therapist will look for opportunities within the session to help the group recognize and defuse from thoughts. She anticipates that these in-the-moment examples will help her group understand how thinking can function and how relating to thoughts differently can help loosen their grip. These experiences will also provide her with opportunities to point to the distinction between Thinker and thought.

Helping the Group Learn to De-Literalize Thoughts

In chapter 1 we discussed how language acquisition involves developing an understanding of certain relations such as *same as*, *compared to*, *belongs with*, and the like, and how this ability enables us to infer relations between things and to link virtually anything together. Once associations are made, they cannot be erased (try to forget that an "apple" is a "fruit," for example). Here's an example of how this can show up in session:

Therapist: Gina, you've been very quiet today. Is there anything you'd like to share with the group?

Gina: No. (*pause*) I just don't talk much in groups.

Therapist: What is it about groups that makes you not want to talk?

Gina: I just don't think I'm very interesting… I don't like to be judged.

Somewhere along the line, Gina learned the concept called "interesting" (and conversely "not interesting"), learned that "not interesting" = "bad," and then linked together "not interesting" = "me" = "bad." Of the many ways a therapist could work with something like this, we suggest a *less* helpful approach would be to respond with "You need to stop thinking that way, Gina." This is because Gina doesn't have the ability to throw some switch and stop these particular thoughts from showing up. Similarly, responses such as "Don't worry, we won't judge you" or "But you've had *lots* of interesting things to say!" can also fall flat.

Understanding language processes helps clarify why this is so. We see that certain associations have been established via relational framing (e.g., *I'm not very interesting, being judged is bad and I can't tolerate that*). We then understand that combating the thoughts, extolling Gina not to have them, for example, or countering them with positive statements is unlikely to work. Further, we can see how these sorts of maneuvers can actually make things worse by just extending the relational network (e.g., *I'm not supposed to have that thought, I should view myself more positively*).

In contrast, let's explore some other therapist responses that might prove more productive. For example, the therapist might choose to simply validate Gina:

> *Therapist:* I'm really glad you shared that, Gina! Those kinds of thoughts can be pretty painful, that you don't have anything interesting to say.

There is a lot happening in these two statements. Empathy is conveyed, of course, and Gina learns that she was heard by the therapist looking through that ACT lens. By pointing to this as an experience Gina is having, the *content* of her thoughts (whether or not she is interesting, whether or not others are judging) has been potentially undermined. The therapist is de-emphasizing the content of the thought, and the way in which the thought functions for Gina may subsequently be altered. Gina's thoughts were left as is, with the therapist subtly pointing to the fact that Gina shared in group despite having feelings and thoughts about not wanting to. The therapist focused on what Gina was doing (versus what she was thinking) and pulled for other aspects of her experience—what Gina was feeling when she was having the thought about not being interesting. This promotes the process of acceptance/willingness discussed in the previous section, as well as the ability to contact the present moment, which we will be exploring shortly. In fact, all the ACT processes are being pointed to here (including self-as-context, values, and committed action), although the therapist has yet to explicitly introduce them. In short, this simple intervention can strengthen key abilities and pave the way for others.

Another helpful response to Gina's comments might be to solicit feedback from other group members:

> *Therapist:* Gina, you took a risk in sharing that. I wonder if anyone else in the group has had that experience—worries about being uninteresting or of being judged.

This response is ACT-consistent, as these sorts of thoughts and worries are treated not as abnormal or as something to be fixed, but rather as a part of being human. Rather than trying to fix notions around needing to be perceived as interesting, or that being judged is bad, the content is left alone as members are guided to consider their larger experience. In this way the processes of contacting the present and acceptance/willingness (and, as we will be discussing, self-as-context) are facilitated. Defusion is promoted experientially. That is, as the group members then talk about their experiences with these sorts of thoughts, the group as a whole undermines the content of the thoughts themselves. Members are defusing from the thoughts by looking at them rather than operating from them. They are effectively undermining the verbal rules that tend to show up with these sorts of worries, such as *I'm not going to speak up since I'm uninteresting* or *I'll be judged and I can't handle that.*

Intentionally watching thoughts is typically a novel way of relating to them for many members. There is an important distinction, however, between being able to notice their thoughts and understanding that what their minds hand them might not be literally true. Gina might be able to notice the thought *I'm way too depressed to do that today*, but if she still buys it she remains in its thrall. The language piece in ACT is important, for it helps the group members understand how they can develop such thoughts in the first place. They are guided to see that such thoughts, while "real" in the sense that they are produced and felt, are often not *literally* true.

When the therapist responds to a thought as an experience (e.g., "So you had the thought that things were never going to change… Did you notice what emotions showed up with that?"), the content of the thought is de-emphasized. The therapist is treating the thought not as a literal truth that therefore needs to be addressed and fixed, but rather as part of a larger experience to be had. Note again that this can be done at multiple levels. For example, working with one member on defusing from a particular thought provides a learning opportunity not only for that member but for others in the group as well. The therapist can also work at a meta-level with the group as a whole: "Has anyone noticed how caught up we've all been in problem solving for the last several minutes? Let's just pause for a moment and notice what our minds are handing us right now."

An important feature of the following exercises is that they alter how language functions. The exercises provide group members with an opportunity to directly experience that change in function, to notice how their relationship with words can shift. It becomes harder to relate to words literally when they can be experienced so differently.

The defusion exercise called Lemon, Lemon, first presented as Milk, Milk, Milk (Hayes et al., 1999), is an ACT standby. (You can find this in the Supplemental Exercises at http://www.newharbinger.com/23994.) It's a standard for us, as it quickly yet effectively demonstrates the different ways language can function. More specifically, it shows us how effortlessly we can create a powerful virtual experience using words, and it also reminds us that in the end, we are just making sounds. Like so many ACT exercises, the group setting really enhances the exercise. With languaging in particular, group members see for themselves how language binds the human experience—how it enables each one of us to do what we do and also how it leads to the suffering that comes with being human.

Experiential exercises such as Silly Voices and Lemon, Lemon provide an opportunity to discuss the role of languaging directly with the group. We create an opportunity for the group to experience a shift in how language functions, paving the way to talk more explicitly about languaging itself, how it works, and how we humans can relate to language in unworkable ways. The following discussion is a version of a dialogue loosely based on the Bad Cup metaphor introduced by Hayes et al., 1999, and detailed in Westrup, 2014:

Therapist: Let me give you an example of this language thing. (*moves and stands beside an arm-chair in her office*) We've all agreed to call this a chair, correct? (*group indicates agreement*) We could have called it something else. For example, in France we would call this chair a "chaise." (*members nod*) But that's just arbitrary—we've all just agreed to call this a chair. We could just as easily call it a "thark." In fact, let's do that. Let's agree that this is a thark, okay? So now I could run into you next week, even next year, and say, "Have you bought any tharks lately?" and you would know what I mean! (*group laughter*) But isn't that something? We take this ability for granted, but look what we've managed to do in less than a minute. We have created a whole new term for this object, and a meaning for the sound "thark"—it means this object now (*pointing to chair*).

Therapist: (*continuing, now stroking the fabric of the chair*) We've also agreed to call this stuff "fabric," and this (*touching a leg*) "wood." Again, we could have called it something else, but we've agreed to call the stuff with these sorts of physical properties "fabric" and the stuff with these sorts of physical properties "wood." (*Group indicates agreement.*) But look what happens if I say to you, "This is the most gorgeous chair in the world." (*Therapist pauses, letting this sink in.*)

*Group
member:*   That's an opinion.

Therapist: Yeah, interesting. It's different, isn't it? "Gorgeous" is not based upon a physical property in the ways "chair" or "fabric" or "wood" are. Gorgeous is more of an interaction between the observer and the object. We can't open up this chair and find gorgeous in there. "Gorgeous" isn't *in* the chair. (*member nods*) But listen to what we do: "I'm inadequate." (*Therapist is deliberately using what has been previously identified in the therapy as the client's most painful thought. For this reason she pauses and lets this really sink in.*) Therapist (*continuing*): Just as "gorgeous" isn't in this chair," "inadequate" isn't in you. We can't open you up and find "inadequate" or "not good enough" somewhere. Just as we can't find the place where "motivation" is supposed to be but isn't. In fact, I can't find "inadequate" anywhere in the universe! Where is it? (*pauses, letting this sink in*) But notice how we relate to those words as though they represent something that is literally real. We relate to them as though they are actually in us as opposed to a concept we've learned to apply to ourselves.

The above discussion pointed to both the power and the arbitrariness of language (e.g., "We could just as easily call it a 'thark'"). We have also directly discussed our tendency to reify language and to relate to the thoughts we produce as being literally true. In her book *Advanced Acceptance and Commitment Therapy: The Experienced Practitioner's Guide to Optimizing Delivery* (Westrup, 2014), Darrah noted that many therapists choose not to explore the role of language so explicitly with their clients and suggests this can shortchange the therapy. Although it can be a little tricky to deliver, this piece can be quite powerful. The day before writing this chapter, in fact, Darrah had a discussion very similar to the one above with a client, a young man struggling with alcohol addiction. A former member of a strict religious sect that taught members that they were bad (evil, in fact) if they did not adhere to the tenets of the church, this client had spent most of his life struggling unsuccessfully with the idea that he was fundamentally bad (for having had problems with the church, for ultimately leaving, for his addiction, and more). As she wrapped up the gorgeous chair discussion with this client, Darrah saw that he was crying:

Darrah: What's happening for you?

Client: (*very choked up*) Bad isn't *in* me!

This notion of "bad," "good," "adequate," "inadequate," and the like being language-based rather than technically in us is clearly an important idea that will be further developed in the self-as-context component of the therapy.

Distinguishing Thinker from Thought

The interrelatedness of the core processes in ACT becomes increasingly clear as we move through the therapy. Contacting the present moment from a stance of willingness, noticing and defusing from thoughts—all these abilities work together and enhance one another. All pave the way for building awareness of Thinker as distinct from thoughts. Members come into contact with the Observer Self, an Experiencer who can bring awareness to the present moment, who can choose to be willing, who can notice thoughts as thoughts.

Simply inviting the group members to observe their thoughts during a mindfulness exercise points to the Observer Self. While not talking specifically about self-as-context, the therapist guides the group to an experiential awareness of being distinct from thoughts. In the Leaves on a Stream meditation exercise, for example, members are instructed to "stand on the riverbank" as they put leaves on a stream and watch them float downstream. What is implied here, through experience, is that while they have thoughts, they are distinct from their thoughts.

As session 4 draws to a close, the therapist mentally runs through the key points she wanted to convey regarding defusion (e.g., looking at rather than simply from thoughts, de-literalizing thoughts, distinguishing Thinker from thought). Her sense is that group members demonstrate reasonable comprehension and that they will have many opportunities to continue to develop their skills through between-session practice and throughout the rest of the therapy. She has been able to pull in experiential learning opportunities that seemed effective. She decides to end the session and asks group members to spend at least a few minutes each day observing their thoughts.

What to Do When Abilities Vary

We turn now to an issue that is an inherent aspect of group work—the disparate abilities of group members. The ACT model is particularly helpful here. Because the core processes are interrelated and interwoven through every session, members will have many opportunities to develop their individual abilities. The therapist can move her group forward without fearing she will leave members behind. For those members ready to learn more, she can introduce and work on additional core processes. However, the processes already introduced will continue to be present throughout, providing the therapist many opportunities to help members develop their abilities. In fact, the therapist is enabled to maximize the vicarious learning available in a group setting, as members will be modeling for one another and it all will apply.

Of course that doesn't mean we always move on! Choosing to work with a very stuck individual can be instructive for the same reasons just mentioned—that whatever process is being worked on will still apply to all members (there is no mastery here). It is highly likely that whatever the individual is struggling with (e.g., unwillingness, fusion with thoughts) applies to the others in the group to some degree. *Function* can again guide you here. How is the group member's avoidance, for example, functioning in the session? Would working with it now serve to illuminate things, or would it result in the group as a whole becoming stuck? Is whatever is happening a manifestation of the very processes being discussed? The answers to these questions form hypotheses that then suggest a way forward. Let's look at an example from session 4:

Therapist:	(*noticing that Dan seems tense, crossing and uncrossing his arms and sighing*) Dan, I'm wondering what is showing up for you right now. What's going on?
Dan:	You mean, what am I thinking?
Therapist:	Yeah, okay. What sort of thoughts are going on for you?
Dan:	I'm just not in a good space today.
Therapist:	That's a thought you're having—that you're not in a good space?
Dan:	I'm not in a good space.

Therapist:	What is that li–
Dan:	(*interrupting*) I've had a bad day. My boss is such a jerk!
Therapist:	Hmmm. So it sounds like you're dealing with those sorts of thoughts, that your boss is a jerk–
Dan:	(*interrupting again*) He *is* a jerk.
Therapist:	And can you see that's a thought you are having about him?
Dan:	It's not a thought, it's the truth.
Therapist:	(*nodding understandingly*) Yeah, this is where it gets kind of tricky. This isn't so much about truth, whether your thoughts are 100% accurate, 90%, or 10% accurate—whether your boss is, or isn't, a jerk. It's about being able to notice the thoughts you're having, to look at them as something that shows up for you at certain times. Even now all of us here are having thoughts about this discussion. Can anyone catch one and share it?

Here the therapist is utilizing the group as a means of learning. She has stepped slightly back from the one-on-one discussion, eliciting participation from other group members and using the collective experience as a learning mechanism. This move also helps her refrain from getting into a right/wrong struggle with Dan—she noticed that he dug in a little as she attempted to help him defuse from his thoughts about his boss. Her hope is that by making the discussion more general, Dan may be enabled to understand what she is getting at. It may take many such interventions before Dan begins to defuse from his thoughts. Regardless, it is likely that the group as a whole learned from this exchange.

Clinical Considerations in Working with Defusion

Process versus content: The work of defusion is all about looking at process rather than content. The focus is on the flow of experience, not the content of the thoughts. Thoughts are held as objects of interest, not as truths that need to be addressed, fixed, or handled in some way.

Timing: Remember that the therapist has been paving the way by frequently modeling this ability throughout the therapy: "I just *had the thought* that I'm struggling with this and not being very clear. Can I ask whether this is making sense to you?" Similarly, from the start of the therapy the therapist has worked to help group members observe their own thoughts. Simple questions such as "And what thought came up when that happened?" or reflecting back, "So it sounds like you had the thought that you weren't good enough" are subtle yet powerful interventions. It has been our experience that group members frequently begin to talk in this way long before defusion is explicitly discussed. That is, they will begin to say things like "Well, first I had the thought that my wife was a nag, and then I realized I was starting to get worked up." Such a client might not yet fully understand the implications of what he just said: that for a moment, at least, he is looking at the thought rather than from it. He might not yet realize that doing so offers him greater flexibility. Nonetheless, he has begun to make an important shift that we can appreciate by simply comparing the differences in the sound and feel of "My wife is a nag" with "I had the thought that my wife is a nag."

That said, we like to get defusion on the table pretty quickly in our ACT groups. The main reason for this is the degree to which thinking tends to dominate behavior. It is very hard to behave in new (value-driven) ways when buying one's thoughts about why that isn't doable. The ability to experience the self as larger than thoughts, feelings, and sensations will remain out of reach if one is lost in the thought process itself. This is why defusion is placed in the first ACT pillar, the ability to be open, as it helps paves the way for the rest of the work.

Explicit versus nonexplicit intervention: This clinical consideration goes hand in hand with decisions around timing. We have pointed out how the therapist has been working with defusion nonexplicitly from the beginning of the therapy (e.g., "I'm *having the thought* that..."). Now, it is time to target this process more explicitly. We do this by providing psychoeducation and generating discussion about the process of thinking, about looking at rather than from thoughts, and about the role of language in thinking.

Experiential versus didactic learning: As with all the core processes, the point is doing, not just understanding. As our therapist demonstrated, we utilize modeling, pointing out in-the-moment examples of thoughts that arise in session, mindfulness exercises, and other experiential exercises geared toward observing and defusing from thoughts.

Summary

In this chapter our therapist tackled the tricky phenomenon known as thinking. While recognizing the powerful influence of thinking in the lives of her group members, she also brought it to ground—revealing the role of language and helping her group members relate to their thoughts in a way that doesn't stand in the way of their living. She took a run at it from three different angles: (1) as a process they can observe, (2) as a product of languaging as opposed to literal truth, and (3) as a phenomenon that is distinct from the Thinker. To accomplish this, she pulled liberally from all ACT has to offer: in-the-moment work, straightforward discussion, metaphors, and mindfulness and other experiential exercises.

Although much practice will likely be required before her group members can defuse from thoughts with ease, they now know what is required and our therapist determines they are ready to move on. In the next ACT pillar, the group will encounter two core processes that will help them more fully comprehend what all this offers. Let's head in now to the centered pillar of ACT.

CHAPTER 7

Contacting the Present

The focus of this chapter is on *contacting the present*, the first of two core processes that compose the centered pillar of ACT. We have examined how acquiring language results in a verbal virtual reality that then overshadows other aspects of experience. In short, our thoughts come to have incredible pull. They pull us into a past that no longer exists to the point that we spend days, even years, reliving unpleasant moments and wondering how things might have been different. They pull us into the future, with the result that we worry and stew about events that have not yet happened (and that may never happen). Even our present is so colored by predictions, evaluations, categorizations, and interpretations that we miss the only moment that is actually ours: *right now*. In ACT we aim to increase contact with the present moment. We want to increase awareness not only of the internal experiences that are occurring (thoughts, feelings, physical sensations), but also of what is taking place in our physical environment. We want our clients to be able to fully contact the present with all its vitality and richness (and yes, its pain).

In this chapter we follow our hypothetical group as members build upon what they have been learning by defusing from thoughts. The therapist has helped them observe their thoughts as an ongoing process, and she will now bring that awareness to other aspects of their experience. We will see how she utilizes exercises that develop the ability to contact the present and how she talks explicitly with her group about this ability. She will continue to seize in-the-moment opportunities to help members build their skills and begin to understand the increased flexibility this brings. They will learn to bring awareness to the very act of being aware, and will begin to understand what approaching life from this stance might offer. We will wrap up this chapter as the therapist paves the way for the second process in the centered pillar, self-as-context.

Putting Contacting the Present into Action

As our therapist plans for her fifth group session, she considers the group's overall progress in the therapy. As a whole, the sessions are active and engaging—all members are participating in the group exercises and discussions. She is noticing a developing ability with willingness as members increasingly choose to head into, and sit with, discomfort as it arises. She has observed that nearly all members have revealed an ongoing control strategy from time to time. Barry, for example, recently commented that if he could just "figure out how to be less self-conscious," he would start going to the gym. This phenomenon is consistent with the therapist's previous experience with providing ACT, which is that the control agenda never completely goes away. Her strategy is therefore to point to the desire to control or avoid discomfort when it shows up, and to highlight such moments as opportunities for willingness. She has some evidence this has been effective as group members are increasingly able to recognize when they are trying to control or avoid discomfort. Moreover, in most cases this noticing has been followed by a move toward willingness.

In terms of defusion, group members are demonstrating the ability to notice and articulate the thoughts they are having, and they are starting to relate to their thoughts as something to be experienced rather than fixed (or blindly followed). All these abilities need further developing, but the therapist feels the group has a good enough start with these that moving forward is appropriate.

For this part of the therapy, the therapist has the following specific objectives: (1) make sure group members first understand—verbally and experientially—what is meant by the term "contacting the present," (2) build their ability to flexibly direct attention to all aspects of experience, (3) help them come into contact with the behavioral freedom that comes with being present, and (4) point to the locus of perspective that is doing all the noticing (experiencing self-as-context). Let's expand on these objectives:

1. Contacting the present: The therapist aims to help the group become aware and *lean into* the moment as it unfolds. This continues to build willingness and undermines verbal rules around what is and is not okay to experience (i.e., defusion). She wants to make sure members understand that contacting the present is *not* another control strategy—as though one is learning to somehow float above the vagaries of life, noticing but not feeling. She will guide her group to notice and fully experience the emotions that show up, and to notice and fully experience various sensations in the body. Contacting the present includes awareness of one's actions and those of others—to track what is actually happening in one's immediate environment (which may have little to do with what one's mind is saying!).

2. Flexible directing of attention: The therapist wants her group to perceive the ability to intentionally direct one's attention where one chooses as a goal in itself. Mindfulness practice as viewed in

ACT, for example, is not in the service of becoming relaxed or achieving some other state. Rather, it is to build the ability to flexibly direct attention to the thoughts, feelings, and physical sensations of the moment.

3. Behavioral flexibility: Just as they are learning to relate to their thoughts differently, group members can also hold even very painful emotions or uncomfortable sensations in a way that frees up their behavior. The therapist hopes to help her group understand that they can notice—and fully experience—the thoughts, feelings, and sensations going on while *doing* what works.

4. Noticing the Noticer: The therapist pointed to the distinction between Thinker and thoughts while working on defusion. As she conducts experiential exercises that develop the ability to contact the present, that distinction will be extended to the Experiencer who is having the experiences of life (including not only thoughts, but feelings and physical sensations as well). This will position the group well to work on the next core process, self-as-context, which we address in chapter 8.

Session Strategy. The therapist will open session 5 with a mindfulness exercise that focuses on contacting the present. She plans to generate a discussion about the exercise, providing an opportunity to assess members' understanding of what contacting the present means and to provide further psychoeducation as needed. She would like to spend as much time as possible in the session practicing, and she has several experiential exercises in mind. Her hope is that as the session unfolds, members will report experiencing some benefits of being present, and she will be looking for opportunities to highlight these (e.g., a sense of vitality, authentic connection, behavioral flexibility). For homework, she will assign practicing today's mindfulness exercise throughout the week. As she assesses her group near the close of the session, she will determine whether or not to head into self-as-context in session 6.

Developing the Ability to Contact the Present

The therapist welcomes the group and moves immediately into a mindfulness exercise. She does the exercise along with the group, not only to support the idea that she is right alongside them in this business of being human, but for practical reasons as well. That is, doing the exercise along with the group helps her with the timing and content of her verbal cuing as she guides the group through the meditation. (For an example exercise, see Contacting the Present Mindfulness Meditation in the Supplemental Exercises at http://www.newharbinger.com/23994.) As usual, our therapist checks in with her group following the exercise:

Therapist:	Let's talk about that exercise a bit. Were you all able to follow along with me? (*Members nod.*) And what did you notice as you were engaging in that exercise? [*Notice the therapist's wording here. She is not asking, "How was that for you?" or something similar that pulls for an "It was good/bad/fine" type of evaluation. Rather, she is pointedly asking what they experienced during the exercise. Her demeanor, too, suggests she is expecting them to be actively noticing their experience—she looks directly at the various group members, clearly waiting for a response.*]
Mary:	It was hard! I don't think I'm doing it right.
Therapist:	Is that a thought you were having during the exercise: *I don't think I'm doing it right?* Or did it show up just now?
Mary:	(*thinks*) Both. I was thinking it during the exercise, and then when you asked the question.
Therapist:	And the thought was, *I'm not doing it right?*
Mary:	Yes. I try, but it's just not working.
Therapist:	Hmm. What do you mean by "not working"? [*Here the therapist addresses content. That is, she could continue to help Mary track what she experienced in the exercise, asking, for example, "Did that thought also show up during the exercise?" However, she suspects that others in the group had similar experiences and that highlighting this might be prudent. Her question is geared to pull out more such content so she can work on it with the group as a whole.*]
Mary:	I can't relax. I try but my mind just jumps off into other things.
Therapist:	(*to group*) You know, my mind was jumping around a bit too today. Was that going on for others as well? (*Most members nod.*) I'm curious, did anyone else in the group have a similar thought show up? About not doing it right? (*Several members raise their hands. Therapist nods in a "Yep-that's-what-minds-do" sort of way.*)

With these last remarks, the therapist is aiming to help members develop their ability to notice their experience and is also furthering defusion by suggesting that this is what minds do. In fact, this simple intervention points to contacting the present, willingness, defusion, and as we will soon see, self-as-context.

Therapist:	(*turning back to Mary*) And then what happens? That thought, *I'm not doing it right,* shows up... Did you notice what showed up next? [*The therapist continues to help*

Mary—and the group vicariously—build the ability to track what unfolds moment to moment. The therapist is guiding Mary to track what she was experiencing during the meditation, and will tie that in with what she is experiencing in the present moment as they are processing this together.]

Mary: I get mad at myself. And then I just give up.

Therapist: Ah, yes. So mad shows up, then you stop… Can you remember what happens next? Like, how do you feel after you make the decision to stop trying? [*The therapist takes the opportunity to emphasize choice, in other words, that thoughts aren't causal. That is, the thought didn't make Mary stop. She had the thought, then chose to stop.*]

Mary: I'm mad at myself. I'll never get this stuff.

Therapist: Hmmm, that sounds painful… I wonder, is that showing up for you right now? (*Mary nods. Therapist nods compassionately and sits silently for a bit, providing an opportunity for Mary and others in the group to simply notice and hold what's in the room.*)

Therapist: (*eventually continuing*) So let's see if I've got this right. You've noticed that as you try to be mindful, you aren't relaxed… Does your mind hand you something about that? Like how you're supposed to be relaxed?

Mary: Exactly. (*raises voice*) Like, *Come on Mary, relax!* (*Mary suddenly laughs along with the group, realizing how this sounds.*)

Therapist: (*laughing as well*) Yeah—I'm gonna try that. Everyone, on the count of three I'm going to tell you to relax, ready? (*increasing her volume on each count*) One…two… three…RELAX!!! (*laughter*)

Therapist: An important thing to see here is that mindfulness isn't about relaxation. Relaxation may show up at some point, maybe not. Mindfulness is about noticing what *is* there… about noticing what's there to be had *without defense*. It sounds like what was there for you, Mary, was the experience of your mind jumping around a bit, the desire and effort to relax, thoughts about what it meant that you weren't relaxing, feelings of being mad at yourself, and so on. It sounds like on the one hand you *were* noticing what was going on for you, and on the other you got caught up in all the commentary your mind was handing you about the exercise.

Mary: Yeah, I was.

Therapist: (*to group*) Is this sounding familiar to you all? (*Members immediately nod.*) Yeah, me too. It's important to see that mindfulness would include noticing *that*. That is, just as we're not trying to force in some experience, like relaxation, we're not trying to get our minds to stop handing us stuff. We want to develop our ability to notice thoughts as part of the experiences going on in the moment.

Mary: I get it.

Therapist: Sometimes people think that "noticing without defense" means "noticing without being bothered." This is yet another way to try to force in an experience, rather than simply noticing what *is*. So, you might notice, for example, that you are feeling tense, and that your mind then hands you an immediate judgment about that. You then have a reaction to that, for example feeling frustrated. We're not trying to have that feeling be gone either, so much as to notice *that* response as yet another aspect of your experience in the moment.

In this intervention, the therapist has clarified for the group what is and is not meant by mindfulness in ACT. She has helped them experientially contact being present to experience and track what they are experiencing. Even as she discussed the content of what Mary shared, she kept one foot in the present. That is, she helped her group members attend to what they had experienced during the exercise while also attending to (and guiding them to also notice) what was showing up during the discussion.

If she wished, the therapist could have elected to take the group through another brief mindfulness exercise as a way to punctuate the points made during this discussion. Our therapist feels that for now the group has grasped things adequately and prepares to move to a different exercise.

Building Flexible Attention

The ability to intentionally direct attention to different aspects of their experience will help group members develop the central objective in ACT—psychological flexibility. As members are increasingly able to defuse from their thoughts, their ability to attend and respond to other information is increased. Let's use our hypothetical group member, Gary, as an example.

Our therapist noted early on that Gary seemed attached to being right. As she has worked with him, she has developed a hypothesis that for Gary (thanks to that relational framing), being wrong = being stupid = being less than = being not okay. She hypothesizes that his interpersonal behavior in the group is often in the service of these learned verbal rules—in other words, he makes sure he is right so that he is essentially "okay." If the therapist is correct, then Gary's behavior is self-reinforcing.

That is, he makes sure he follows the rules (remains okay by being right), so they are never disproven and continue to govern his behavior.

The therapist has been helping Gary learn to notice his thoughts in such moments, such as, *I am having the thought that I am right about this and need to prove it*, or, *I'm the only one who knows what I'm talking about*, or, *Dan is trying to show me up and I need to win.* She hopes to alter how such thoughts are functioning for him so that they are not rules that must be followed but something to be noticed. At this point in the therapy she is helping Gary expand his awareness to other things besides what his mind is handing him, such as emotions and sensations (e.g., *I feel pressured, anxious, keyed up*) and what is actually happening around him (e.g., Mary is looking bored, Gina looks anxious, Dan is acting as though he wants to end the conversation).

When possible, she has solicited feedback from the group to strengthen this sort of tracking, as in her comment, "Dan, I'm wondering what you experienced with Gary during that interaction just then." The aim is that this expanded awareness will help Gary learn to take what his mind hands him with a grain of salt. He might recognize the consequences of his behavior rather than being dominated by the verbal virtual reality in his head. He might become increasingly aware of the distancing effect his behavior has with others in the group, for example. He might try a new behavior (e.g., "Okay, I can see your point") and notice its actual versus preconceived consequences (e.g., Dan looks pleasantly surprised and hasn't said anything to "get him," other group members are smiling, he is still "okay").

Benefits of Being Present

In her initial session, the therapist had mentioned to her group that a goal in ACT is "vital living." As members have moved from avoidance to willingness, as they have learned to defuse from their thoughts and increase contact with the present, they have likely begun to taste the vitality that comes with living in the present. Now our therapist wants to gently bring attention to some benefits they might experience from engaging in life in this way.

Therapist:	Dan, I'm wondering what came up for you just now as you were talking about your daughters…
Dan:	I just worry about them, you know?
Therapist:	Yeah, I do know! It seemed like you got in touch with something just now…(*waits*)
Dan:	(*struggling with himself a bit*) It's just hard… (*Therapist is silent, Dan eventually continues*) I just really care about them, you know (*suddenly choked up*). (*The therapist is in no hurry, just sitting with Dan and the other group members as he contacts his feelings.*)

Therapist:	(*nodding respectfully*) That is clear. In fact, let's just honor that for a moment (*models settling in to the experience*). Let's just notice and hold what is showing up right now. (*Therapist closes her eyes in order to better contact the emotions in the room, and Dan and others in the group do the same.*)
Therapist:	(*continuing with long pauses between cues*) Notice the worry and the fear…notice how you can actually lean into it, this fear that you carry for your daughters…notice the profound love for them right alongside the fear… Lean in now, see how fully you can experience this stuff. (*The therapist is silent for a few moments as Dan does this. Allowing herself a quick check around the room, she sees that a tear is running down his face, and that others in the room appear moved. She then continues.*) Notice that it's all there, and that we can hold it all. We can hold our worries and our fears in a way that lets us be present to the good stuff too. Love, joy, connection…this, right here—this is the fullness of life. (*Therapist sits silently with them for a bit longer, then wraps up the exercise by inviting Dan to take a couple breaths and thanking him for being willing.*)

The therapist senses that this exercise was impactful for the group. Members seem moved, thoughtful. She decides that this is one of those times when the exercise speaks for itself and any verbal processing might actually detract from the experience. She does have a bit more time left in the session, however. She decides to do another quick exercise that also points to the increased information available when we bring our attention to the present. This exercise, Noticing the Room (Benefits of Contacting the Present), can be found in the Supplemental Exercises at http://www.newharbinger. com/23994.

Distinguishing the Experiencer from the Experiences

Our therapist wishes to only lightly point to the idea that just as there is a distinction between Thinker and thought, there is a distinction between Experiencer and experiences (e.g., one is not a thought but rather *has* a thought; one is not anxious but rather *has the experience* of anxiety). She knows this will be expanded upon as the group moves into the self-as-context core process, so she does not spend much time discussing it in detail. Rather, she seizes opportunities such as the following:

Mary:	I was so depressed over the weekend! All I could think about was how I am wasting my life.
Therapist:	Was that thought hanging around the whole weekend?

Mary: Pretty much. I mean, there were moments where it wasn't there I guess…but I didn't want to do anything!

Therapist: Bear with me Mary, while I work with you on your language a bit. I recognize that this was a painful experience for you. But I'm wondering if you can talk about it in the way we've been discussing in here. Remember how we talked about how we *have* thoughts, rather than we *are* our thoughts?

Mary: Yeah. So…I had the thought about wasting my life.

Therapist: Exactly! That's a tough thought to have no doubt—tough emotions come with it, but it's still an experience you're having.

Mary: Yes, I see that. It seems better somehow. Not better, but…less big or something.

Therapist: Using our words in this way reminds us that we are not these painful thoughts, we experience them. We're the Thinker, not the thought. (*Mary nods.*) And it's not just thoughts. All the emotions that showed up, the physical feelings…those are also experiences to be had. We're the Experiencer, not the experiences.

The therapist is pleased with the group's participation in today's session. Based on their behavior during the exercises and the comments they've made throughout the session, she feels members have at least started to develop the ability to contact the present. She is most pleased by their increasing ability to be present to what naturally shows up during the session and by some comments they've made that indicate they are intentionally choosing to be present despite some discomfort going on.

At this point the therapist is tempted to move a bit into self-as-context, but she is also thinking of a guided imagery meditation that she suspects would be powerful for this group (the Tonglen meditation, which can be found in the Supplemental Exercises at http://www.newharbinger.com/23994). There is not much time left in the session, however, and there's no need to rush things. She also senses that group members have learned plenty for one session and might want to just ponder things for a bit. She decides to end the group a few minutes early. Before closing, she invites them to continue what they were working on in today's session:

Therapist: I'd like to encourage you all to experiment a bit with what we were doing today. That is, see if you can really get present from time to time, noticing and watching your thoughts, noticing the feelings and sensations showing up. See how fully you can notice and experience your world as you move through it…just as we really got present to this room for a few minutes today and came into contact with all sorts of things that were just waiting to be noticed and felt. See what else might be waiting in your world, ready to be *really* seen, ready to be *fully* experienced.

Clinical Considerations in Working with Contacting the Present

Process over content: We have found it easier to refrain from getting pulled into content when working on contacting the present, simply because the focus of the work is so clearly on noticing (rather than answering, addressing, solving). We do take care to specifically point out that contacting the present is an ability—there is no destination here.

Timing: Similarly, viewing contacting the present as a skill guides us in terms of when and how to introduce mindfulness practice. It is useful to begin with shorter, more basic mindfulness exercises, moving to longer exercises—including guided imagery meditations—as members' skill level increases. We also assign daily mindfulness practice between sessions and regularly check in with members regarding how this is going.

Explicit versus nonexplicit intervention: All along, the group members are learning to contact the present. Modeling and highlighting in-the-moment experiences (e.g., thoughts, feelings, sensations) helps the group members increase their awareness of the flow of experience. At this stage in the therapy, we tend to talk more explicitly about what we are doing.

> *Therapist:* I'd like to start off with a mindfulness exercise. I'm going to be asking you to direct your attention to different things during the exercise—for example, I might invite you to notice your thoughts, then I might ask you to notice whatever emotions are showing up. I might have you notice your body and whatever physical sensations might be there, sounds, smells, the temperature of the room. The key is to notice that we can do that—we can put our attention where we choose from moment to moment.

As more and more core processes are explicitly discussed in the group, earlier exercises and metaphors can be revisited as a way to draw a thread through the therapy and tie things together.

> *Therapist:* Do you remember a couple weeks back when we did the Eyes On exercise? (*Members think a moment, nod.*) That's an example of what we're doing here. That is, your minds were going *crazy* in that exercise, telling you all sorts of things about it. Your bodies were sending you all sorts of anxiety signals, you were giggling, sweating…the works. And yet, you were also able to direct your attention to the present moment, to the exercise you were participating in. You were able to direct your attention to your partner, even with all that going on. That's pretty powerful stuff.

Experiential versus didactic work: At this stage of the therapy, we can move easily from experiential work to didactic discussion about the core processes being targeted (e.g., willingness, defusion, contacting the present). In some cases it is useful to spell out what an exercise is geared to illustrate before doing it with the group—highlighting key points in advance can often facilitate the group's learning. At other times, it is effective to move straight into an exercise so that the experiential learning will speak for itself. (There is no right or wrong—we do our best to assess the current context and make the best decision we can. Should it seem that an idea or exercise is not being received as intended, we can always change course by bringing in another exercise or talking about what is happening with the group.) The experiential work is continued by modeling being present to the group and by making space for members to do the same (e.g., not filling space with words, simply allowing moments to be).

Summary

In this chapter we followed our therapist as she and her group members explored contacting the present. It was essential to begin with clarifying what is meant by this core process in ACT, and the therapist addressed this directly and also by conducting exercises that provided opportunities to practice contacting the present. She emphasized the flexible, intentional nature of directing one's attention in this way and helped her group members contact some of the benefits that come with living in the present. She pointed to the Experiencer, who has thoughts, feelings, and sensations (but is distinct from those thoughts, feelings, and sensations). In essence, she highlighted a process she has been developing from the start, talking about it explicitly and facilitating experiential learning. She is ready to head into the next core process in the centered pillar—self-as-context.

CHAPTER 8

Developing Self-as-Context

In this chapter our group will work through the core ACT process known as *self-as-context*. The abilities fostered in this part of the therapy are instrumental in the development of psychological flexibility. Consider the challenges of being willing, for example. The therapist has introduced willingness as an alternative to battling unwanted thoughts, feelings, or sensations. But what a thing to ask! It's not a stretch to imagine that some members of her group have had moments of such despair that they no longer want to live. We can guess that at least one member's day-to-day experience is colored by self-loathing; perhaps another carries memories so painful the merest hint of them brings nausea and panic. Even in her own life, the therapist contacts fear or pain only to immediately shy away. Why on earth, *how* on earth, would her group members choose willingness when what's there to be had is so darn hard?

The ability to experience self-as-context offers a place on which to stand, an immutable sense of self that is not threatened by even the most painful thoughts, feelings, and sensations. In this chapter we will demonstrate how the therapist helps the group contact this way of experiencing the self. As discussed in chapter 1, there are three aspects of self-experiencing that are of interest in ACT: self-as-process, the conceptualized self, and self-as-context. In the following sections we will see how our therapist guides her group through these distinct but related processes. She will talk explicitly about the ability to experience self-as-context, but she will also be relying on in-the-moment examples and experiential exercises to help members' abilities progress.

Putting Self-as-Context into Action

The therapist has been looking forward to working on self-as-context with her group. Her experience has been that when group members fully comprehend and experientially contact this piece of the therapy, it is a game changer. She also knows, however, that it is usually the most difficult core process to learn. She feels her group is ready, especially due to members' increasing ability to defuse from thoughts. (In her experience, if a group member is still unable to notice and look *at* thoughts, he or she will have difficulty accessing self-as-context.) The therapist has allotted at least two sessions to work on self-as-context and is prepared to spend additional sessions focusing on it if needed.

Session Strategy. The therapist plans to open session 6 with another mindfulness meditation that guides the group members to direct their attention to different aspects of their experience. (In the interest of space, however, we will not provide it here; instead, please see the Building Flexible Attention meditation in the Supplemental Exercises at http://www.newharbinger.com/23994.) She wants to use this exercise as a platform to tie willingness, defusion, and contacting the present more explicitly to the ability to experience self-as-process, which then opens the door to exploring self-as-context. Her plan for the majority of this session is to address these two aspects of self-experiencing, self-as-process and self-as-context, through discussion and experiential exercises.

The therapist has the following objectives for session 6: (1) continue to build the ability to experience self-as-process, (2) facilitate flexible rather than rigid attachment to the conceptualized self, and (3) build members' ability to contact self-as-context. Below we consider these objectives more closely:

1. Experiencing self-as-process: The group has been developing this ability for some time. Learning to notice and defuse from thoughts and learning to attend to what one is experiencing in the moment both require the ability to experience self-as-process. The therapist intends to continue to draw the group members' attention not only to what they are experiencing in the present, but also to this noticing ability itself. She plans to point to this during the mindfulness meditation and other experiential exercises, and as in-the-moment opportunities arise.

2. Flexible attachment to the conceptualized self: The therapist aims to help her group members view the various concepts they have of themselves as just that—concepts they have learned via language, and then learned to attach to themselves as identities. We will take a moment now to clarify what she is hoping to accomplish, using some hypothetical group members.

The therapist has worked with her group for a while now and has noticed various ways in which members self-identify. For example, Dan sees himself as a "screw-up," Gary is a "tough guy," and Gina sees herself as "person who doesn't matter." What's more, she has observed how these various conceptualizations appear to influence behavior: Dan doesn't contact his children because he's sure they have no desire to interact with "the screw-up," Gary doesn't share feelings that reveal his vulnerability, and Gina rarely speaks up in group or in her life more generally.

These conceptualizations are the products of relational framing. Certain associations had to be made before the concept called "screw-up" held any meaning for Dan, for example. Somewhere along the line he learned to relate "screw-up" with being "bad" (a concept that also had to be learned) and then to apply that "bad" "screwup" categorization to his self-identity. Remember that once made, these associations can't be unlearned (try to forget that "apple" is a fruit). Adding to the difficulty, our minds are geared to efficiently seek "coherence"—evidence that supports previously made associations. In other words, we see what we look for. If you have ever tried to forcibly change or correct someone's thinking, the following exchange may sound all too familiar:

Dan:　　　　I'm such a screw-up. My kids don't want anything to do with me.

Mary:　　　　You're not a screw-up!

Dan:　　　　I *am*! I really screwed up with my kids.

Therapist:　　You were trying as hard as you could.

Dan:　　　　No, not really. I could have done a lot more.

Therapist:　　You are working hard to be there for them now…for example, you just helped your daughter out with that car payment–

Dan:　　　　(*interrupting*) If I was a better father, she wouldn't *be* in that situation.

And so on. Fortunately what we have learned about relational framing offers our therapist another way to work with the various notions of self that are keeping her group members stuck. For example, rather than try to get Dan not to have the thought about being a screw-up, she can help him view that thought as a behavioral product, something he has learned to produce. In short, the therapist can help her group members hold their notions about themselves more lightly. Dan can carry the thought of being a "screw-up" while *being* with his kids in the way he envisions a "good father" would be.

It is important to note that in ACT we aren't concerned solely with "negative" self-concepts. Rather, we aim for flexibility—the ability to hold these ideas of ourselves lightly enough to respond to life effectively as it unfolds. For example, a group member could have developed an identity based on achievement that has served her well in many ways (e.g., *I am smart and good at things*). However, it could also function as a barrier if rigidly held (e.g., *If I fail it means I have no value*).

Another important point is that our therapist is not aiming for group members to not have self-concepts (as if she could!). Rather, she hopes to help them hold their identities in a way that is workable given what they're up to in their lives. The next aspect of self-experiencing, self-as-context, greatly facilitates this process.

3. Experiencing self-as-context: The ability to experience self-as-context is an inherent part of experiencing self-as-process and learning to hold the conceptualized self more lightly. In other words, both of the latter processes point to the Noticer who is noticing what is unfolding—that locus of perspective that tracks one's experience through time.

Just as the therapist helps group members learn to notice and defuse from thoughts, she aims to help them "notice who's noticing" the thoughts (or feelings or sensations). She wants to help the group members recognize that all their various notions of themselves, from being "not okay" to being an "Achiever," are distinct from the Experiencer (or Noticer) who is aware of such conceptualizations. There is an important implication here. If that awareness—that locus of perspective—is distinct from the internal phenomena of the moment, and that awareness has also been constant through time as various thoughts, feelings, and sensations have come and gone, it must be more than, larger than, all those thoughts, feelings, and sensations. Even if one's experience has been rife with thoughts of worthlessness and feelings of being broken in some way, the awareness itself of such experiences is, and has always been, intact. What a thing to come into contact with!

Experiencing self-as-context opens the door for group members to fully engage in their lives in a way that is workable for them. It is no longer necessary to wait until the right sorts of thoughts and feelings come along in order to live as they would like to be living. This is the psychological flexibility the therapist is aiming for in this therapy.

As we observe our therapist as she moves through the objectives listed above, we will see how interrelated they are. That is, furthering self-as-process furthers self-as-context and vice versa. Experiencing self-as-process and self-as-context can help group members hold even longstanding conceptualizations of themselves in a more flexible way. So while the selected exercises and metaphors in this chapter might highlight a particular aspect of self-experiencing, they are actually relevant to all three ways we conceive of self-experiencing in ACT.

As planned, the therapist opens session 6 with a mindfulness meditation (see examples in the Supplemental Exercises at http://www.newharbinger.com/23994) and then processes the exercise. Given her planned focus for the session, she looks for opportunities to make a distinction between Experiencer and experiences ("Mary, when you had the thought that you were antsy, what else showed up?"). She is now poised to move through the key points regarding self-as-context.

Loosening the Grip of Self-as-Content

The therapist has been working on helping group members hold their identities more lightly from the outset of therapy. To clarify, the "content" in self-as-content refers to all the categorizations, evaluations, and interpretations that members have learned to apply to themselves. The therapist's deliberate use of language has helped members contact the distinction between *being* all that content and *having* (and noticing) all that content. Earlier the therapist might have simply reflected back to Dan, "So you're *having the thought*: I'm a screw-up." Now she will point more explicitly to the processes involved (because previous sessions have put these processes on the table).

Dan: I can't get over being such a screw-up with my kids! I start thinking I make progress, and then something happens. Yesterday–

Therapist: (*interrupting*) Let's just take a moment and notice what's happening. Settle into this moment with me, Dan. (*Both fall silent for a moment or two.*)

Therapist: (*continuing*) So what are you experiencing right now?

Dan: I feel bad. I feel like—I'm having those thoughts again about being a screw-up.

Therapist: Great catch Dan! You just caught that you were in the thoughts and pulled back enough to notice them, to look *at them*. (*Dan nods.*) We've talked about how being able to look at our thoughts in this way helps us remember that we aren't the thought, we *have* the thought. It sounded like you were also noticing other stuff, like a "bad" feeling—do you mean the feeling of sadness?

Dan: Yeah, I have sad feelings, guilt. I'm mad at myself. (*Therapist looks at him, and he quickly corrects himself.*) I'm *having* the thought that I'm mad at myself, the feeling of being mad… (*Both sit silently for a bit, as does the rest of the group.*)

Therapist: (*continuing*) And if I remember correctly, this is when "I'm a screw-up" tends to show up.

Dan: Oh yeah, that's there big time.

Therapist: Yeah. That one has been pretty predictable—we almost expect it to show up with stuff like this. (*Dan nods. They both sit silently for a bit as they consider this. The therapist can see that the other members of the group are listening intently.*)

Therapist: (*to Dan*) Notice how you are there, and I am here, (*to rest of the group*) and you all are there, and we're all noticing and watching what shows up for you at times like this. (*lets this settle in for a bit before continuing*) It sounds like something similar happened yesterday…

Dan: Yeah, my daughter wasn't list-

Therapist: I'm so sorry to interrupt again Dan, but I'm wondering if we could do something here. That is, I've no doubt that something upsetting happened yesterday and I'm not suggesting that doesn't matter. But I'm wondering if you can do the same thing you were doing just now; simply speak to what you were experiencing at the time. What was going on for you?

Dan: (*thinks*) I was mad, scared—

Therapist: You were *having* the feelings scared, mad…

Dan: Yeah, and I was having thoughts about my daughter not listening. Then I yelled, then I had the thought of being a screw-up, then I felt—had feelings about being guilty…

Therapist: Great Dan—what you were just able to do isn't easy! It's especially hard when you're in it, right? It's when our thoughts are most troubling—sometimes we say it's when we have the "stickiest" thoughts—that it's hardest to notice them as thoughts, as something that is showing up. Have you guys noticed that? (*to the rest of the group members who readily nod*) Dan, can you imagine for a moment that you were in the situation with your daughter, and whatever was rolling out with her was rolling out, but you were able to stay present with your experience? That is, imagine you were there, actively noticing the thoughts and feelings going on as something that was showing up for you…do you have a sense of what that would be like?

Dan: (*thinking it over*) I think I would be less reactive, less mad. I'd handle it better for sure.

Therapist: Okay, this is important: "Mad" is part of what you're experiencing—

Dan: (*interrupting*) I get it. I would be *noticing* feeling mad…but I still think I'd be handling it better.

Therapist: (*really emphasizing this as she speaks to entire group*) Okay, you are really onto something here. Mad would be there, and notice how it doesn't have to go away! Something about being able to notice it as it's there, as something you're experiencing, though, would free you up to *act* in a way that sits better with you. (*Group is silent, taking this in.*)

Therapist: (*to Dan*) And notice how the thought *I'm a screw-up* could be there in full force. There you are…*I'm a screw-up* shows up—

Dan: But I don't have to *be* a screw-up. (*Tears start in his eyes as he contacts the import of this. The therapist nods meaningfully; she is also a little emotional and makes no attempt to hide this. She sits silently with the group, modeling leaning into the moment.*)

The previous exchange points directly to values and committed action, but the therapist knows she will be heading there soon with the group and is content to let things stand. She explicitly pulled out the ability of experiencing self-as-process and included conceptualizing oneself as a screw-up as part of that process. She then helped Dan and the others in the group see how willingness, defusion, contacting the present, and experiencing self-as-process might look when applied to real-life situations.

A strength of group work is that it provides a means to develop what is sometimes referred to as perspective-taking ability. When group members learn to view themselves from different perspectives (provided by group feedback), they are aided to view themselves less rigidly. In other words, they are less firmly attached to self-as-content. Consider the following exchange:

Therapist: Gina, I notice you have not said anything today. At times it looked to me as though you started to say something, but then you stopped. Was that going on for you?

Gina: I guess so.

Therapist: (*waits*)

Gina: (*eventually*) Like I just don't have anything to say, nothing that matters, anyway. I stop myself because I realize there's no point.

Therapist: So, you have a thought, something you want to put out there, but then you have the thought that you don't have anything important to say so there's no point.

Gina: Yeah.

Therapist: And can you tag anything else? In that moment, when that thought shows up about not having a point, what emotions are there?

Gina: Sad, I guess. I'm afraid.

Therapist: So sadness is there, fear as well…

Gina: Yeah.

Therapist: And what about now? What are you experiencing as we talk about this? [*Again, the therapist is working on willingness, defusion, contacting the present, self-as-process; we see how interrelated these abilities are.*]

Gina: Same thing…sad… I wish people cared what I had to say.

Therapist: Yeah. It is not hard to understand why that might be a sad, even scary experience. If I were in your shoes, wanting to participate but having thoughts about it not mattering and people not caring, I'm sure I would be feeling sad and afraid. [*Here the therapist is working on perspective taking. That is, she is certainly validating Gina's experience but in a way that invites Gina to look through her (the therapist's) eyes. Though the type of thoughts might be the same, Gina is nonetheless considering the therapist's perspective of her (Gina's) situation.*]

Therapist: (*looking around at the group*) I'm wondering what you all are experiencing right now as you hear Gina talk about this. [*Now the therapist is inviting different perspectives. As Gina listens, she is provided a window into how her experience is viewed through the eyes of others. She also gains perspective on aspects of others' experiences that may not have been obvious from where she is sitting.*]

Mary: I feel frustrated. Because I do want to hear from Gina and I feel like she doesn't trust us enough to tell us what is going on with her.

Stan: I actually feel the same way lots of times. Like people don't care what I have to say, or that what I'm saying is stupid or something.

Gary: I feel like that *after* I say something, like, *I can't believe I just said that. Now they're gonna think I'm an idiot...*

Therapist: Yeah, I have that one too! And of course I always think about what would have been *better* to say. (*Several members chuckle and nod.*)

Barry: Well, I don't see that in Gina. I mean, I know she feels that way about herself, but if I didn't know that, it wouldn't have occurred to me. I actually think she has lots to say that is important. But I know me saying that probably doesn't change anything...

Therapist: Isn't that something! We all have these virtual realities in our heads about ourselves...it's a wonder we can do anything at all! (*Group members, including Gina, chuckle and nod.*)

There is a lot happening in this exchange. Rather than Gina being limited to the self-concept her mind seems to hand her in moments like this (e.g., that she is a person who doesn't have anything to say) and conceptions about others (e.g., they are people who don't care), Gina now has information that contradicts or certainly extends this sort of thinking. It is helpful to remember that the therapist is not looking for Gina to suddenly see herself as a person worth listening to, as though now her thinking has been "corrected." The associations she's made around herself and others have been made and can't just be erased. They can be added to, however, as she now has new information, different perspectives about her participation in group. Perhaps most importantly, Gina was guided to attend to the actual context she is in—not just the verbal virtual reality in her head. She may find there are often times when she has something meaningful to say and that others are actually listening.

This discussion of why and how to develop perspective taking is in fact light treatment of a complex topic; hopefully we've shown enough for readers to get a sense of how this ability pertains to the self-as-context piece of ACT. We would like to think that therapists who have been conducting groups might begin to see why certain interventions create positive change—what it is, for instance, about certain types of group feedback that furthers psychological growth—and apply this to refine their interventions in ways they find useful. We direct those interested in learning more about how to apply RFT principles in their therapy sessions to the (masterful) *Mastering the Clinical Conversation*, by Villatte, Villatte, and Hayes (2015).

Developing Self-as-Context

So far in session 6 the group has participated in a mindfulness meditation followed by a general discussion that led to further exploration of experiencing self-as-process, including noticing and holding one's self-concepts lightly (illustrated in the dialogues above). Our therapist now wants to home in on helping her group members build their ability to experience self-as-context.

She has spent some time pondering what seems to make this part of the therapy so clinically significant and arrived at three key ideas she would like to get across to her group: (1) recognition of the distinction between Experiencer and experiences, (2) recognition of the self as whole and intact, and (3) recognition of the ability to choose regardless of thoughts, feelings, and sensations.

The therapist is going to rely on experiential exercises and metaphors now, using group discussion only to underscore and clarify certain points. In other words, she isn't going to try and "teach" experiencing self-as-context. The main reason for this is that experiencing self-as-context isn't just a concept to grasp, it's a felt experience. It is also an experience that is typically quite foreign for group members. It's heady stuff—all this business about self-experiencing, self-concepts, being whole—and yet it carries huge potential for meaningful change. The therapist decides to do an exercise that is active and typically very engaging, a nice balance to the introspective work that's gone on so far.

The Timeline
(self-as-context)

The therapist has come to the session prepared for this exercise. Specifically, she has brought a string (roughly twelve feet long), pens, and a small pad of sticky notes. (She could also use yarn, index cards, and pieces of paper cut in half.)

The therapist has all of the group members recall around five or six major events that occurred in their lives. Common examples are marriages, deaths, divorces, graduations, and moves. However, she also encourages them to recall a small moment in time that had great impact, such as "the first time someone said 'I love you' to me."

Using one piece of paper per event, she has each member take a piece of paper, fold it in half, and write just a few words about the event on half of the paper. She asks for a volunteer from the group to share his events. Dan volunteers.

The therapist then asks Gina to hold one side of the string. This will represent the moment of birth. The therapist stands about eight feet away (it could be less if space is limited) and holds the other end of the string, representing the present moment. She makes sure there is some length of string left over (the reason will be explained shortly).

She asks Dan to place the first chronological event on the string (timeline) in the proper place (between birth and the present), depending on his age when it happened. She instructs him to discuss that moment in time in as great detail as possible, including what was particularly important for him about this occasion. Group members often gloss over the details, but she encourages Dan to drop into the moment deeply to harken back as much as possible. The therapist interjects comments such as "sounds like a beautiful day" or "I imagine that was very painful," but she avoids processing each moment in time for too long. Instead, she invites Dan to move to the next event.

Once he has placed the final event on the timeline and has detailed the experience, the therapist asks Dan to stand right next to her. She says, "So, you have shared with us some of the major events in your life, and you have revisited those particular days. At the beginning of the rope, Gina represents the day you were born, and here you are with me, standing at the present moment. Looking down the timeline of your life, there is a connection between the moment you were born and now. We look at your life from this view (holding her arm away from her body so Dan can see the pages hanging from the string), where the contents of your life are clearly visible, or from this view (holding the string up to his nose), where you see the common thread of life leading back to birth." (This demonstrates the difference between looking at your self-as-content and self-as-context.)

The therapist can also use this exercise to point to the opportunities that lie ahead—paving the way for the values work to come. That is, she can turn so that she is facing away from the past (the string with all the cards on it) and ask: "What else do you notice about this?" (pointing to the extra string pooling at her feet).

Dan: There's lots of string left.

Mary: Lots of life to be lived! And notice how our minds want to fill all this in (*waving her arm around the air in front of her*)—it wants to tell you all about the future based upon the past (*pointing to the cards*)! But here *you* are (*indicating the string at the present point*). The future is unwritten, and *you* get to decide how you're going to move through this life.

This exercise has many advantages, particularly in a group setting. It is active and engaging, and it provides a tangible demonstration of self-as-context (and of possibility). Members benefit from looking at another's life from this perspective, and it can be done with as many group members as the therapist wishes. In fact, our therapist would like to spend the rest of the session on this, and she has just enough time to run through the exercise with another group member.

Session 6 is drawing to a close. The therapist is feeling pretty pleased with how group members are working with self-as-process, and she believes they are beginning to understand how their self-identities are also something to be noticed. Now that these ideas have been discussed and worked on a bit, she can continue to tie them in throughout the rest of the therapy.

She believes the work has begun on self-as-context as well, although, as to be expected, some members seem to have greater understanding than others. Barry, for example, has been quieter than usual and has not appeared particularly struck by the exercises or group discussions, and the therapist suspects Mary may not be understanding as much as she seems to (she has noticed that Mary engages in therapist pleasing at times). She will be keeping an eye on both of them as she continues to work on self-as-context in the next session. For now, she feels the group has done its work for the day. She again asks members to continue their daily mindfulness practice throughout the week, bringing particular attention to the Noticer who's doing all the noticing.

Strengthening Self-as-Context

We hear repeatedly in our supervisory, training, and consulting experience that the self-as-context piece is the most difficult aspect of delivering ACT. It is also typically the piece that clients find most challenging. We think this is fitting. We are peering at consciousness itself and attempting to use the very tools that color our awareness to do so (meaning language processes). If you have the experience of your brain folding in on itself, you are not alone!

The therapist was happy with the group members' work during session 6. Since the Timeline exercise went so well, she did not finish with as thorough an explanation of self-as-context as she had intended. Therefore, she believes session 7 should be spent further developing self-as-context and is prepared to spend the following session on this as well if she determines the group is not where it needs to be at the end of session 7. She will continue to monitor Barry, as he was unusually quiet after the exercise, and Mary, as her pleasing agenda often masks her ability to understand what's been presented. She wants to make sure all her members (1) understand what is meant by the "Self," and (2) develop the *ability* to experience the self-as-context. How will she approach these objectives?

1. Understanding what is meant by the "Observer Self": The therapist has pointed to the Noticer, to the Experiencer, and so on, but she wants to do some double checking around how members are understanding this term. (By the way, it is likely she will never use the term "self-as-context" in her group, as it is not very user-friendly, but will use terms such as the "Self" or the "Observer"—all in reference to awareness itself, that locus of perspective that is constant and that moves through time.) She will use metaphors and exercises to help illuminate this way of experiencing self-as-context and will also explicitly discuss what is meant by the term "Self."

2. The ability to experience self-as-context: The therapist is aiming for the group members to bring their awareness to—to experientially contact—that locus of perspective that is always there, larger than, and yet in contact with, the experiences that come and go. Once they have a sense of what is meant by self-as-context, some sense of what it's like to experience the self in this way, she will continue to develop their ability with this core process.

Session Strategy. The therapist plans to begin session 7 with a guided meditation, Observer You (Hayes et al., 1999), which is designed to bring attention to self-as-context. This meditation guides the group through various experiences members have had through time, bringing awareness to the locus of perspective that runs throughout and is larger than those experiences.

The therapist would like to follow the Observer You meditation with an experiential exercise called the Label Parade (Walser & Westrup, 2007), which provides a physical representation of the distinction between internal experiences (e.g., thoughts and feelings) and the Experiencer. An active exercise, it would serve as a nice counterbalance to the long meditation the group will have just completed. It can take up a great deal of time, so the therapist will be careful to leave enough room to introduce her favorite ACT metaphor, the chessboard. She has consistently found the Chessboard Metaphor to be powerful in her ACT groups, as it simply does a great job of illustrating self-as-context in a clear and accessible way. She hopes that ending the session with it will help bring the idea of an intact, continuous self home. The Chessboard Metaphor, which has been extensively covered in the ACT literature (e.g., Hayes et al., 1999; Walser & Westrup, 2007; Westrup, 2014), uses various chess pieces to represent the content of group members' lives (experiences, thoughts, feelings, sensations, memories) and a chessboard to represent the context that holds—and yet is distinct from—those experiences.

As she had planned, the therapist opened session 7 with The Observer You exercise. (A detailed description of this exercise can be found in the Supplemental Exercises at http://www.newharbinger.com/23994.) The therapist is always careful to assess the group's experience following the meditation and usually finds that responses vary. We have witnessed those ranging from lukewarm reactions to game-changing epiphanies such as "I've been there all along!" It can be helpful to remember that no one exercise, metaphor, or discussion is *the* mechanism for change. That is, if a particular intervention doesn't seem to resonate for a group member, rest assured there will be plenty of other opportunities to further the core processes you are hoping to develop. We don't need to convince or persuade a group member to "get" a particular exercise if it just doesn't seem to be working for her. We have also observed that interventions that don't seem to bear fruit in the moment can nonetheless take hold and burst into bloom at a later point in the therapy. Remember, too, that one member's struggle with a particular exercise or metaphor can create a powerful learning opportunity for others in the group.

She is now checking in with the group:

Therapist:	Was everyone able to contact the "observing, continuous you"? That "you" that has been there through all those experiences?
Barry:	(*looking doubtful*) I didn't really get that. I don't know what you mean by the "Self" or the "Observing Self."
Therapist:	Well, let's try something. Are you aware that you're sitting in that chair?
Barry:	Yeah.
Therapist:	And could you hear yourself saying, "Yeah"?
	(*Barry nods.*)
Therapist:	Could you feel yourself nodding just then?
	(*Barry nods again.*)
Therapist:	And can you notice certain thoughts going on for you right now? And maybe some emotions?
Barry:	(*pauses a moment*) Yeah.
Therapist:	That you that is noticing is the Observing Self. That's the "you" that knows you're sitting there in this moment and that knew you were having an experience this morning. (*Barry nods in comprehension.*)
Therapist:	Sometimes we tend to think this is harder than it is. What I mean is that we over-think it, we strain to "find" the self rather than recognizing the awareness that is already there.

As she assesses the reactions of her group members (Mary is nodding, as though she suddenly understand this now), it seems to her they are getting it. The therapist wants to capitalize on this momentum, so she moves straight into another experiential exercise, The Label Parade (Walser & Westrup, 2007), which can be found in the Supplemental Exercises at http://www.newharbinger.com /23994.

Our therapist suddenly looks at the clock and realizes she is completely out of time. She had planned to do the Chessboard Metaphor, but it will have to wait. She reflects that perhaps it's for the best. This last exercise seemed to go extremely well, and the reactions of her group members lead her to conclude that she should let the implications of the exercise just sit for a while. She is also very aware that the ability to experience self-as-context is both foreign and challenging (given the pull of those sticky thoughts); revisiting and strengthening self-as-context in the next session by introducing the Chessboard Metaphor would likely serve the group well.

Clinical Considerations in Developing Self-as-Context

Process over content: It can be said that self-as-context is all about not being our content! We are deliberately strengthening group members' ability to see that they are not all their content (thoughts, feelings, sensations), but they have and experience content. Self-as-context is the very process of attending to the distinction between process (that awareness that is constant yet moving through time) and content (all that awareness notices and holds).

Timing: It's interesting to consider the timing of when to work on self-as-context. On the one hand, that way of experiencing the Self is always there, always available. On the other, thanks to languaging we tend to be stuck in our thoughts and out of touch with the self that is larger and intact. What this means in terms of clinical decision making is that the therapist can choose when to illuminate what is always there. If time was very limited, for example, our therapist might point to this process directly very early on. (As we have seen in these chapters, she has instead developed it more indirectly, reserving explicit discussion for the *centered* portion of the therapy). It is quite possible that someone could have a sudden epiphany around self-as-context that would illuminate what all the other processes bring.

If we have the time, we prefer to approach self-as-context gradually but steadily, devoting several sessions to working on it. A sequential approach to the therapy paves the way, allowing members to create space (willingness), get unstuck from the cognitive ticker tape (defusion), get present to their experience (contacting the present), and direct attention to different aspects of experiencing (self-as-process). Ultimately, they arrive at contacting the awareness itself (self-as-context).

Explicit versus nonexplicit intervention: Timing plays a major role in whether or not self-as-context is developed explicitly or by less explicit methods. Again, by explicit we mean to clearly call out the ability, to point to it as a process. Our example therapist never actually used the term "self-as-context" but did begin to call it out as the "Observing Self," the "Noticer," and the "awareness that is larger than." She began, however, with more subtle references (e.g., "What else are you experiencing?"). Early comments such as "So what else showed up with that thought?" gradually evolved to "Notice the You that is experiencing this moment, a you that is larger than these moments that come and go." Once this important ability is named and group members understand the process it entails, we can move freely between explicit and nonexplicit interventions to continue to strengthen their skills.

Experiential versus didactic work: Of course experiential work is key with all the processes, but particularly so when words are inadequate. Just as experiential learning helps individuals who are very fused with thoughts get unstuck from them, such exercises help members experience a sense of self that is definitely not about words.

Summary

In this chapter we have followed our therapist over two sessions as she developed self-as-context in a group setting. In actuality, our therapist began the work at the outset of therapy by using language that helped the group develop the ability to notice self-as-process. She eventually targeted this ability more directly in session 6. She then extended that awareness to noticing the Noticer, highlighting the distinction between that awareness and the internal phenomena of the moment. She looked for opportunities (e.g., using peer feedback) throughout the therapy to help group members look at themselves and their experiences from different points of view and hold their self-conceptualizations in more flexible ways. Finally, she moved into developing the ability to experience self-as-context, drawing upon metaphors and experiential exercises specifically designed to pull out these processes.

Helping a group develop this piece has significant impact. Once members contact the self that is larger than thoughts, feelings, and sensations, things begin to shift. Even the most painful experiences can be held in a different way. Unworkable, rigid notions of the self are seen as things that have been learned. Old reasons, explanations, and conclusions as to why life isn't working no longer stand, and more, may no longer be necessary.

At this point in the therapy our hypothetical group has moved through two of the three ACT pillars: open and centered. Now that the processes of willingness, defusion, contacting the present, and self-as-context have been explored and are in play, our group is ready to move to the third and final pillar: engaged.

CHAPTER 9

Working with Values

O ur group has moved through the open and centered pillars of ACT and is poised to begin working with values (the first of two processes composing the engaged pillar of ACT). Group members have learned how to be fully present from a stance of willingness: noticing while not necessarily buying the thoughts of the moment, noticing and simply holding the emotions and sensations that arise. They have learned that that they are fully capable of this sort of experiencing, that they are in fact larger than, and distinct from, the internal phenomena that come and go. All this begs an interesting question: if thoughts and feelings aren't in charge, if in fact we don't need to fix them or avoid them or wait for them, on what *do* we base our actions? Values, as conceived in ACT, offer a direction in which to head.

In this chapter our group will wrap up self-as-context and work through values. When she determines it is time, the therapist will introduce valued living as an option to the group, carefully defining what is meant (and not meant) by "values" in ACT. She will assist her group members to identify their personal values in different life domains. She will then clarify the difference between values and goals as viewed in ACT and will help members develop goals that take them in the direction of their values. Next she will explore with the group some of the barriers that often stand in the way of valued living. As usual, she will be doing this work by means of psychoeducation and group discussion, and by introducing relevant metaphors and experiential exercises. We join our therapist as she plans for session 8.

When she first laid out her strategy for this ACT group (see chapter 4), the therapist allowed for the possibility that self-as-context might require more than two sessions. Even though the last two sessions targeting self-as-context have gone well, she is hesitant to move forward. She wants her group members to have a solid understanding of this core process and to come into contact with the gifts of experiencing oneself in this way (i.e., as whole, intact, 100% acceptable). She decides to continue with self-as-context at the start of session 8 and, depending on her assessment of the group, either head into values or continue developing group members' ability to experience self-as-context.

Session Strategy. The therapist will open session 8 with a mindfulness exercise that speaks to self-as-context. She will then check in with the group, assessing members' reactions to last week's session and how their daily mindfulness practice is going. She will be assessing the group's understanding of self-as-context throughout this discussion. For example, when learning about members' experience with their mindfulness practice, she will inquire whether they "noticed the Noticer" and generate a discussion about self-as-context as it pertains to mindfulness practice.

Next, she will introduce the Chessboard Metaphor, described briefly in chapter 8 and presented in detail in the Supplemental Exercises at http://www.newharbinger.com/23994. She will take her time with this, allowing for as much group discussion as needed. She thinks it might work nicely if she can introduce values at some point in the discussion—perhaps near the end when she demonstrates that the chessboard can move in a direction while carrying all the chess pieces. She is prepared to move more explicitly into a discussion of what is meant by values in ACT, and she will bring Clarifying Values Worksheets (Walser & Westrup, 2007) for the group to complete before the next session.

Rather than detail the objectives for the values work she plans to do, we will immediately join the therapist as she begins session 8. We'll return to values as she heads into that core process.

Wrapping Up Self-as-Context

The therapist welcomes the group and completes a mindfulness exercise. She then shares a little about what she experienced during the Timeline and Label Parade exercises in the last session, stating, "There were a couple of points where I had chills! I was really moved by what went on in here last week." She wants to (a) help the group reconnect with their last session, and (b) generate a discussion that helps her assess where her group members are with self-as-context overall. She then conducts the chessboard exercise.

As hoped, this metaphor was powerful for the group. There was much discussion afterwards, and several members were emotional as they contacted what it means to be (and to always have been) whole and 100% acceptable. The therapist finds herself wanting to linger here. Although she did point to valued living when demonstrating that the chessboard could move in a direction while carrying all its pieces, she is reluctant to head into anything new. What's showing up in the room is rich.

Accordingly, the therapist simply allows the conversation to continue, modeling leaning into the emotions that are showing up. Eventually, the conversation slows. Looking at the clock, she sees she's got a bit of time left in the session. She could end it here...perhaps there's another exercise she could do... Suddenly she remembers a guided imagery meditation (The Mountain Meditation, revised from

Kabat-Zinn [1994]; found in the Supplemental Exercises at http://www.newharbinger.com/23994) that does a beautiful job of pulling out self-as-context. She decides it is perfect timing to do this with the group.

The therapist feels strongly that any processing following the Mountain Meditation would take away from it. She is pleased with the session and notes a lot of emotion in the room. She doesn't want to diminish this with *any* more talking, in fact, so she simply thanks the group and encourages them to "bring today's work with [them] throughout the week."

From everything she was seeing and sensing in the last session, the therapist believes that the main objectives she wanted to convey to her group around self-as-context have landed. Primarily, members' reactions to the Chessboard Metaphor were what she had hoped to see. They were all visibly moved, very thoughtful, almost wordless as they came into contact with this way of experiencing the self. She is pleased that now that they have come into contact with the awareness that is always there, it will be easier for them to reconnect with this way of self-experiencing. She intends to help them with this, pointing to the Noticer and "Self that's larger" whenever possible. For now, the group is ready to head into the next core process, values.

Putting Values into Action

Session Strategy. The therapist will open session 9 with a mindfulness exercise that creates an opportunity for the group to experience self-as-context. She wants to pull that process into the room again and intends to strengthen it as much as possible throughout the remainder of the therapy. Next, she will move into working on values. Although she has pointed to values throughout the therapy, now it is time to explore this topic more explicitly and help her group articulate values in various life domains. She is allowing plenty of time for psychoeducation and also has a Clarifying Values Worksheet she will hand out and go over in the session. Based on her experience, some members may require only some values clarification—understanding values as meant in ACT—while others may need help contacting what they truly care about. The worksheet will assist with this and will help members distinguish between values and goals.

The therapist has identified four objectives for this core process, which are to help group members (1) understand the meaning of "values" as defined by ACT, (2) identify core values within various life domains, (3) learn to develop goals that are in the service of values, and (4) identify and overcome barriers to valued living. Let's explore these objectives more closely:

1. Values as defined in ACT: The therapist will help group members understand that valuing in ACT is about choosing what to stand for in their lives. She will help them articulate what is important to them and how they want to be in the world. "Living according to one's values" is not about arriving at some destination, however, as though one wakes up one day and crosses "being loving" off the list. Valued living is a choice made over and over again. So, values as conceived in ACT are never attained, but rather serve to guide one's choices.

Our hypothetical group members entered therapy either to fix themselves or because they were waiting for something (or someone) in their lives to change. They have been living in reaction, as though they have no choice in the matter. By being guided to articulate and intentionally choose their values, they will have the opportunity to experience what they do day to day as an expression of those values. As they identify what is important to them in their heart of hearts, they may come back into contact with dreams and desires they have forgotten or pushed aside long ago.

2. Identifying and clarifying values: When helping group members develop their values, it is important to identify values that are always immediately accessible to them. Consider, for example, our group member Mary, who says she values "peace and calm." Although there is no "wrong" in valuing these experiences, living in pursuit of this can be problematic. For one thing, along with other emotional states, feeling peaceful and calm requires the cooperation of Mary's environment. Circumstances well beyond her control can interfere (and do)—traffic, work conflicts, annoying phone calls…the list of things that can evoke anything but calmness is endless. For another, pursuing a particular emotional state such as calmness can lead to rigid rules (e.g., *I can't confront my boss; he'd get upset*) and unworkable behavior (e.g., avoiding conflicts to one's detriment).

For these reasons our therapist seeks to help group members identify values that are always within their reach, and that expand rather than limit their options. "Kindness," for example (as long as it is being held as something the group member is doing rather than expecting from others), is always accessible. Regardless of what is going on in the moment, the group member can make a choice that is in the service of being kind.

3. Goals in the service of values: Whereas values can never be attained (like points on a compass, they simply point to a direction), goals as viewed in ACT are discrete and attainable. Once the therapist has helped her group members identify their values in different areas of their lives, she will help them identify specific actions they can take in the service of those values.

4. Barriers to valued living: The therapist would like to identify and work with her group on some of the barriers that stand in the way of living according to one's values. She anticipates this will be a relevant issue for the remainder of the therapy (and beyond) and that as the group moves into committed action, members will be experiencing many of these obstacles.

Defining Values as Meant in ACT

The therapist has alluded to values at many points in the therapy (e.g., "It sounds like being honest in your relationships matters to you"). Now, she wants to enable her group members to articulate for themselves what it is they care about and how they want to be in the world.

Therapist:	We've been working a lot on noticing that we're not our experiences. That is, we *have* thoughts, but we're not our thoughts, we *have* feelings, but we're not our feelings. All that stuff is on our board and we can carry it. In fact, we don't even need the "good" pieces to win! We can have our thoughts and feelings, even the really tough ones, and still be okay. (*pauses*) There is nothing that needs to change; there is nothing missing in us. (*pauses*) That leaves us pretty free.
Gary:	Are you saying we can do what we want?
Therapist:	There will always be consequences, Gary, to everything we do. What I'm pointing to here is that we don't have to wait to be more, better, or different before we can start living the way we want to be living. (*pauses, let's group think this over*)
Therapist:	(*continuing*) So that's the essential question I'm putting in front of you today: who do you want to be in the world? (*let's this sink in, then continues*) What kind of friend do you want to be, what kind of partner? What kind of employee or neighbor? If you don't have to wait for different pieces to show up on your board, if you don't have to move them around anymore…how do you want to be living?
Gina:	I want to be happy.
Therapist:	I'm really glad you said that Gina. Yes, of course you want to be happy. Me too! The thing is, we've talked a lot about what happens when you make your life be about trying to have certain feelings or doing away with others—
Gina:	Oh yeah…
Therapist:	But this is perfect! You are showing how our minds work. We want to somehow figure everything out so that we arrive at happiness. And then we wonder why it isn't working, or what it is about us that keeps it from happening. (*Group members are nodding in recognition.*)
Therapist:	(*earnestly*) Gina, I hope you have many happy moments in your life. But pursuing feeling happy as a goal keeps you digging (*Gina nods, recognizing the man-in-a-hole*

reference). This is about *you* deciding what *you* care about in your heart of hearts. You get to decide how you show up in the world.

The therapist continues to help the group conceptualize values in the ensuing discussion. Once she has the sense that that members understand values as conceived in ACT, she moves into helping members articulate their own values.

Identifying and Clarifying Values

As the therapist just stated to Gina, valuing in ACT is a very personal business. However, a group setting can be helpful for this work. Not only is it comforting for group members to witness their peers similarly struggling with identifying and articulating their values, but it also enables them to get ideas from one another and inspire each other. Our therapist has prepared several questions that tend to generate fruitful discussion around this topic (see below).

Before beginning, she assures the group that not all the questions will be meaningful to everyone in the group. She states that if a particular domain doesn't "speak to them," it's perfectly fine to skip it. She then unhurriedly moves through the following questions, making plenty of space for whatever shows up in the room. Group discussion is welcome here.

1. What do you want…? What do you really, really, really, *really* want?

2. What kinds of relationships would you like to build?

    a. With your friends

    b. With your family of origin

    c. With your partner/future partner

    d. With your child/children (current or future)

    e. With your community

3. What do you dream about doing in your spare time?

4. What would you like your career to look like in your wildest dreams?

5. What do you want your life to stand for?

6. What kind of person do you want to be?

7. What is important about your spirituality?

As she works with the group, the therapist guides them to consider values that, again, are always accessible:

Barry: I just want respect, you know?

Therapist: What does that mean to you, being respected?

Barry: You know, *respected*. Like, people listen to you, don't push you around. (*thinks a bit*) When you're respected people take you seriously…

Therapist: Okay, let's work with this. If I've got this right, being listened to is important, not being pushed around…you want people to take you seriously (*Barry nods*). Okay, bear with me—Can you think of someone you respect?

Barry: (*thinks*) Yeah, my brother-in-law.

Therapist: What do you respect about him?

Barry: He's really…he doesn't play games. He calls it like he sees it, but…he's also fair, you know? People know he means what he says and you can trust him.

Therapist: Is it safe to say that those are things that are important to you then? Not playing games, being fair, meaning what you say, being trustworthy…

Barry: Absolutely. Yeah, I definitely respect the guy.

Therapist: So this is super important. If you make your life be about *getting* respect from others, that means you're only going to be okay if you are getting that from people. And as you know, it's pretty hard to make people feel or act certain ways. But you seem pretty clear on a way of being that *you* respect. A way of being in the world that *is* absolutely within your power. *You* get to decide if you are fair, if you say what you mean, if you behave in a trustworthy way.

Barry: (*thinking*) Yeah. Yeah, I get that. So my values would be those things?

Therapist: This is your call. It only matters if it comes from *you.*

Barry: (*thinking it over*) Yep, that's what matters to me. That's always been what matters to me.

The previous exchange was illuminating not only for Barry but for the others in the group as well. As she continues to work with them, the therapist is looking for values that point to ways of showing up for life, such as engaged, present, loving, open, honest, forthright, kind, trustworthy, compassionate, dependable, accepting, and responsible (notice these are all adjectives that describe behavior). She is careful, though, not to put words in members' mouths. Rather, she helps them unpack values to get at the quality of *being* that matters to them and that is within their power to uphold.

Values on the Whiteboard
(identifying and clarifying values)

The therapist decides it would be timely to do a group exercise geared toward identifying and clarifying values. On her whiteboard, she lists ten different life domains that are often seen in the ACT literature (Hayes et al., 1999): family of origin, intimate relationships, friends, community, caregiving, work, health, education, leisure, and spirituality. She then invites members of the group to go to the board one by one and add their values to as many domains as they wish.

Afterward, the group members examine what has been written on the board and discuss what has been shared. The therapist finds that members are very helpful in assisting their peers to clarify their values.

Therapist:	Barry, this seems difficult for you; I noticed you didn't put any values on the board… What's going on for you?
Barry:	(*hesitates, confesses*) Well, once I write something on this board—something that's important for me—that probably means I have to do something about it.
Therapist:	Ah! So there is a part of you having difficulty with the notion of having to be accountable for your identified values; that you have to behave in a certain way in accordance with your values, all the time, without fail.
Barry:	Yeah! That's it! I mean, if I say that I value my health and commit to changing some of my eating habits and all of you fine people see me walk into group with a cherry Danish hanging out of my mouth, you're all going to know I'm a hypocrite! (*Everyone laughs.*)
Therapist:	(*smiling*) I get that, Barry. If you identify what you want your life to look like and don't do it perfectly all of the time, then you're not doing anything well enough. Does that sound like the chatter in your head?
Barry:	Yeah, sounds familiar but much more nicely said than what's in my head. (*Members laugh.*)

Therapist: Well, what if I told you that you would still be moving toward your values, even if you did a *crappy* job of it? (*The therapist has noted Barry's use of humor in this situation, and she hypothesizes it is a way for him to manage the discomfort he seems to be experiencing. She could opt to work with him on willingness but decides it is more clinically important to stay on task with identifying vales.*)

Barry: Say what?

Therapist: Seriously! If you decide to change your eating habits in order to move toward your value of health and vitality, if you eat salad instead of french fries just *one time* in a week, isn't that bringing you closer?

Barry: Yeah, I guess so, *crappy job*, it is! He writes on the board, "In service of my values of health and vitality, I'm going to change my eating habits to include healthier choices."

Therapist: (*waits for Barry to take his seat amid much applause from the group, then speaks more seriously*): So Barry…(*looking at the board which leads Barry to look at it as well*), how does that feel to look at that on the whiteboard for all to see?

Barry: It's actually a little scary. (*keeps staring at what he wrote, and begins to get a bit emotional*) But you know, it feels great. It feels like I know where I'm going. I might not know how to get there yet, but my health is important to me, and now it's out *there* (*pointing to the board*).

Therapist: Nice, Barry. (*pauses, savoring the moment*) Thanks for sharing what's really important to you with us.

Notice that once Barry came into contact with his value around health, he dropped the humorous banter and contacted the emotions he was experiencing. The result was a meaningful exchange that created an opportunity for real change.

Defining Goals in the Service of Values

Group members are only just beginning to get a sense of how values are approached in ACT and what their personal values might be. Nonetheless, the therapist wants to head into the distinction between how values and goals are conceptualized in ACT. In her experience, there is often confusion between the two, with members frequently treating values like goals (or the other way around), and she wants to clarify this as soon as possible.

> *Therapist:*   We have been working on values and starting to identify the values that are personally relevant to you. I'd like to take a moment to clarify the difference between values and goals. Values are like points on a compass: north, south, east, and west. We don't ever arrive at them. Rather, they point the way. Goals are the specific steps we take in the direction of those values. So Barry, you identified "health and vitality" as being values. Can you identify a specific goal that takes you closer to those values?
>
> *Barry:*   Well sure, like you said, eating a salad instead of ordering french fries one time this week.
>
> *Therapist:*   Perfect! That's a specific goal you can attain that takes you closer to your values around health and vitality. (*to group*) That's the main difference between them. Goals are attainable, values are guiding lights, or points on a compass. We don't wake up one day and say, "Phew! I'm healthy now" and cross it off our list. (*group laughs*) That value, being healthy, being vital, will *always* be there, on days when you move toward it, and at those times when you move away.

The whiteboard exercise and subsequent discussions have taken up most of the session time. The therapist still decides to hand out the Clarifying Values Worksheets and asks members to complete them between sessions. This sheet, available at http://www.newharbinger.com/23994, asks for values in various domains, similar to the exercise the group just completed with the whiteboard. However, it also asks respondents to rate the importance of each domain, to identify specific goals for each, and to list thoughts and emotions that could function as barriers. The therapist considers waiting until the next session to hand out the sheets so she can go over them more thoroughly, but she decides it might be worthwhile for members to make an initial stab at it on their own—wrestling with this stuff is good! She will then use part of the next session to go over these worksheets with the group. After handing out the sheets with a (very) brief explanation, the therapist ends the session.

Applying Values to Daily Life

The therapist's assessment of her group is that all members are in about the same place when it comes to values. There is more work to be done, however. That is, they seem to understand how values are viewed in ACT, and the distinction between values and goals. But they need to spend much more time with this core process, particularly as it applies to their lives and the sorts of obstacles they might encounter. She would like each member to have well-articulated values and clearly specified goals in place before moving into the final core process: committed action.

> **Session Strategy.** The therapist will open session 10 with a mindfulness exercise geared toward identifying values (often called "the Funeral" exercise but originally presented as the "What-Do-You-Stand-For" exercise; Hayes et al., 1999). After processing this with the group, she will ask members to share their experiences with the Clarifying Values Worksheets. She anticipates needing to do a fair amount of psychoeducation as she works with them on these, answering questions and helping them clarify values and identify attainable goals. She will also be looking for opportunities to work with some of the barriers that tend to stand in the way of living one's values. She'd like to end with an experiential exercise, Values in the Trash (a version of the Two Sides of a Coin exercise; Follette & Pistorello, 2007). This has typically been a powerful exercise in groups, underscoring the central point of valued living in ACT.

The therapist welcomes the group, then asks them to prepare for a guided imagery exercise. She then conducts the Funeral exercise as a way to help members contact their values. (This exercise has been detailed many times in the ACT literature, so we will not demonstrate it here. In short, the group members are guided to imagine, at some point in the distant future, their own funerals. They are guided to create this event in the way they would "most like it to be" and to have whomever they would like in attendance. They then are cued to have these individuals speak about how they experienced the group member, and specifically to have this be about how they *ideally* would like to be experienced and remembered by these people. The end result is clarification of how they would like to be showing up in their lives.)

After concluding, the therapist is careful to assess how members experienced the exercise. As has been her experience, a couple of group members had difficulty visualizing their own funeral, constrained by their histories and what their minds handed them about their future. Gina, for example, shared that she didn't have any friends at her funeral—clearly she was unable to create what she wanted for herself "in her heart of hearts." The therapist works with her to see that the very fact she was so saddened by this pointed to what she really wanted and valued—friends who would come and speak to the authentic, caring friend they had in Gina.

The therapist then asks the group how filling out their Clarifying Values Worksheets had gone. As expected, they had struggled a bit, and she spends much of the remainder of the session working on this and assisting members to identify and clarify both values and goals. The therapist also uses this session to explore some of the barriers that members might encounter as they pursue a value-driven life.

How to Work with Barriers to Valued Living

Our therapist knows that a number of factors will arise that will make it difficult for group members to move in the direction of their values. She knows she will be helping them with the barriers that show up as they apply this and start "moving with their feet" (e.g., committed action). However, she would like to point to some of the most common barriers now so that group members can also be on the lookout (and perhaps move through them more quickly).

Avoidance: This barrier will show up again and again as the group moves from values identification to committed action.

Therapist:	*(while watching and assisting here and there as members work on their Clarifying Values Worksheets)* Hey Gary, last week during our whiteboard exercise, you told the group you valued work and what you had to offer as a salesman. You also said that the next day you were set to have a conversation with your supervisor about a new idea that you had—something you thought would increase sales. *(Gary nods.)* How did that go?
Gary:	Well, I left group and I started thinking about the conversation with my boss. Every time I thought about it, I just kept thinking what if he doesn't like it? What if he thinks I'm an idiot with this idea? If he hates this idea, it will just confirm what I've thought all along, that I really don't have anything to contribute to my job. [*Notice the fusion and rules, and conceptualized self.*]
Gary:	*(continuing, laughing a bit but also rueful)* I had a couple of pops of tequila, to be honest, but it did calm my nerves. I'm embarrassed to say that a couple turned into a couple more, and before you knew it, I was waking up with a hangover! So, need-less to say, it wasn't a great time to have that conversation with my boss. *(Gary's acting a little cavalier, but the group can see he's genuinely embarrassed.)*
Therapist:	Wow, I'm sorry to hear that. Sounds like a rough time. Gary, it seems as though the thoughts that you had leading to drinking were really bothering you, so you tried to get rid of them. Is that right?
Gary:	Yeah, I was avoiding.
Therapist:	How great that you see that. And, is it safe to say that the avoiding continued? That is, you had an action, a goal, that you wanted to take in the service of offering your best as a salesman. First wanting to avoid the anxiety, and all the thoughts and feel-ings coming up around the conversation, wanting to avoid how you anticipated your

boss might react and how you would feel about that, avoiding what it would be like to talk to him when you had a hangover, and then…since then?

Gary: Yeah. I've been avoiding ever since.

Therapist: I really appreciate you sharing this Gary. (*to group*) Does this sound familiar to anyone? (*All members nod vigorously, smiling at Gary.*) Yes, avoidance is a biggie. But the first step is recognizing it, as you did. Can you think of what else might have helped in the moment? Let's say, when anxiety showed up, Gary's mind is having a fit, the urge to drink shows up…

Mary: He could notice that and maybe do some mindfulness?

Therapist: Noticing is key. You will find there are days when living your values is more difficult than others. The key is to *maintain contact* with your value, even when the going gets tough.

Gary: (*thinking*) Yeah. I think that if I had "gotten present" as you say, and remembered what I'd said I was going to do, or really *why* I had said I would do it, I might have been able to make a different choice.

Therapist: That's huge, Gary. And that is what this is all about. Luckily our values don't go anyplace. You get to continue to care about what you bring to your work as a salesman regardless—you will always have the next moment to choose whether you will move toward that or not.

Values as means to an end: Another common barrier to valued living is using values as a means to get something (or get rid of something). In ACT the emphasis is on values as an ongoing guide to behavior, not a means to an end. This is a bit tricky, however. That is, it is not a stretch to imagine that as group members live differently (according to their values), aspects of their lives will change. Being able to imagine that future can pull members forward, helping them make value-driven choices even when it's quite difficult. Our therapist will work with her group on these sorts of nuances whenever she can.

Dan: Hey, I wanted to tell you guys that "in the service of my value of being a reliable friend" (*makes air quotes*), I called my buddy Mike and told him he could rely on me to help him move. He told me that since he hasn't heard from me for so long, he assumed I wouldn't be helping him after all, and found somebody else to help. So much for values I guess.

Therapist: Dan, it sounds like that was painful for you. I am wondering, though, did you offer help to your friend to show up as a reliable friend, or was there more behind what you expected from offering to help? [*The therapist is checking for a secondary gain behind choosing this as a value.*]

Dan: Well, I've really been trying hard to change, and it would be nice if people noticed.

Therapist: Hmm, perhaps you were looking to get some validation out of the offer? That would be nice for sure. But remember, valued living in ACT is about how *you* choose to be, not what others do or what you receive from others. (*pauses as Dan thinks this over*) Let me ask you this: can you continue to be a reliable friend because it's something you chose as an important way to show up for your friends?

Dan: I'll keep trying, I guess. It'd just be nice to hear an "atta boy!" every now and then.

Therapist: For sure. It's tricky. On the one hand, it's no small thing to say at the end of the day, today I honored my value around friendship by offering to help Bob move. Notice how that's not about him. At the same time, we can also imagine how your life might change if more often than not, you lived according to your values. For instance, we can imagine what your friendships might look like if over time you can continue to be a reliable friend. (*pauses as Dan and the group thinks this over*) Since that is something you have struggled with in the past, do you think it might change the course of your friendships if you stick with it?

Dan: Well, I sure know which of my friends I can count on, and which ones I can't. (*smiles*) I *would* like to be more like the ones I can rely on!

Here the therapist identified the potential barrier that arises when values are used as a means rather than as a way of being. However, she also drew upon Dan's ability to imagine how his friendships would improve by consistently behaving in a reliable way. Even though this scenario is in the imagined future, Dan can still access the reinforcing qualities of such relationships, which then facilitates moving in that direction. Additionally, by helping Dan identify what he cares about and then have those values be the point (not what he hopes to receive), he gains access to the reinforcement of making value-congruent choices (e.g., "I am offering to help because I value being a reliable friend").

Choosing socially desirable values: A problem can arise when members select values because they are socially desirable. This is often driven by fusion with rules and attachment to a conceptualized self as "good person." This tendency is particularly prevalent in a group setting, so the therapist is careful to check for this. She specifically asks if values are being determined by what members think they "should" be valuing, for example, or because others (e.g., parents, the culture) want them to have the value. This is important as such rules can really interfere with members contacting what is personally true for them.

If a member selects a value that's in the service of gaining approval or being acceptable to others, he is then dependent on others' reactions. That is, a value that is chosen in order to gain favor is only reinforcing if it "works." Remember Dan wanting to be a reliable friend? He was ready to give up on the notion because he didn't get reinforcement from others. The therapist was able to help Dan determine that he really did want to *be* reliable and that he could access this way of being regardless of others' reactions.

Values that aren't reinforcing: Values help members create a "life on purpose" by building the anchors for repeated patterns of behavior that then move them in valued directions. It's hard work. For some domains—which members haven't visited for a while—it's *very* hard work. So, if there isn't a reinforcing quality to behaviors that move them toward their values, the likelihood that they will be repeated is quite low.

This is why the therapist really digs in when helping members identify their values. She wants to determine what the member finds reinforcing about the value, and double-check for intrinsic gains. For example, she asks questions such as "What would it mean for you to show up as a present parent? What would that feel like?" When she hears certain responses that seem heartfelt ("I would be the type of parent I've always dreamed of being"), she knows they have hit the sweet spot of valuing. She moves into the Values in the Trash exercise, which can be found in the Supplemental Exercises at http://www.newharbinger.com/23994.

Once again the therapist wants the experience the group just shared to end on its own. She makes sure she doesn't rush out of it and move on, so she just sits for a bit with the group. It's time to wrap up session 10, so after a minute or two, she simply smiles at her group members and says that she looks forward to seeing them next week.

Clinical Considerations in Working with Values

Process over Content: When working with values, we want to focus on content, helping group members put into words what they want to stand for and care about. This is deliberate, as verbally linking doable behaviors with deeply held values helps members bring awareness to, and make, choices that will be intrinsically rewarding (instead of choices that tend to keep them stuck). However, we also emphasize the overarching process of valued living. Values in ACT are about vital, meaningful living, not arriving somewhere.

Timing: Although values can be brought in at any point in the therapy, our example therapist took her group through ACT in a sequential fashion based upon the open, centered, and engaged pillars of ACT. Values, being in the last pillar, were approached with many of the other processes in play. As we have seen this therapist do, however, we take opportunities to point to values throughout the therapy, waiting until this point to go into them in depth.

Explicit versus nonexplicit intervention: We mentioned that we often seize opportunities to point to values as they occur throughout the therapy. For example, we might comment, "So, being a good dad is clearly important to you," even while waiting to explore that specific value more fully. Once we have explicitly introduced values, we frequently employ terms such as "identifying values," "valued living," and "value-driven choices."

At this point in the therapy, we are pretty free to talk about all the processes as they arise in session. That is, when it seems useful to do so, we point to willingness, looking at thoughts, getting present, and experiencing the Self that is larger. We might even begin to use the words "committed action," although the group has yet to focus specifically on that process. (We feel free to do so because their meaning is straightforward and we are not concerned the term will be confusing or misconstrued.)

We do continue to employ nonexplicit interventions as well. That is, our stance in the room and our responses to the group provide continued opportunities to model and strengthen the core processes. Even if highlighting a particular idea or core process, we likely facilitate abilities in many members. For example, imagine that while discussing her values, Gina shared something very painful. The therapist might continue to help Gina put her values into words, but in simply pausing for a few moments, compassionately sitting with Gina as they contact the sadness of what she has shared, she also furthers willingness and contacting the present.

Experiential versus didactic work: Perhaps more than at any other stage in the therapy, we provide a great deal of psychoeducation around values. It is important to help the group understand what to shoot for in terms of values and why, and how values differ from goals. We work with members as they wrestle to articulate those values, both in conversation and on paper. However, we don't forget the power of experiential learning and utilize exercises such as the Funeral exercise and Values in the Trash to create a felt experience around this key tenet of ACT.

Summary

In this chapter the therapist worked with her group to develop the core process of values in ACT. Over the course of two sessions, she helped members understand both values and goals as conceived in ACT and to identify and articulate their own values. She assisted them to develop discrete, attainable goals in the service of those values and worked through some of the barriers that can stand in the way. She drew heavily upon psychoeducation in these sessions but also utilized metaphors and experiential work to help members contact the fullness and vitality of a value-driven life.

Once this hard work is finished and values and goals are clarified, group members are at a point where it is time to move. None of the work that's come before means much if it doesn't translate into action. A value-driven life is one of purpose and vitality—action is required. The next and final core process, committed action, will bring this to the fore.

CHAPTER 10

Creating Committed Action

Like most of us, our group members can envision lives that would be better if only they did certain things. And like most of us, translating that into action is another matter. Fortunately, just as all the other core processes in ACT can be developed, the ability to take *committed action* is a skill that can be learned. This final core process is in fact essential to psychological flexibility, tying together all the other core processes learned in ACT.

This chapter picks up our group as members learn to make behavioral choices (committed actions) that take them in the direction of their values. The therapist will spend her final two sessions working on this core process, beginning by pulling in the values work done in sessions 9 and 10. She will then work with her members to develop short-, medium-, and long-term goals that are in the service of those values. She will explore barriers to committed action, helping her group learn to recognize and overcome what can stand in the way of making value-driven choices. Finally, we will see how she chooses to conclude the therapy with her group, honoring the work they have done together and paving the way toward a vital and meaningful life.

Putting Committed Action into Action

The therapist's assessment of her group at this point is that members are developing the skills needed to move through life in a psychologically flexible way, and that they now have a direction in which to head (based on their personally chosen values). She is anxious to really get them moving now—they have only two sessions left to meet. She wants to spend today's session setting and identifying goals that reflect the values they've developed, setting them up to practice their skills between now and the final session.

As mentioned above, the therapist has identified two main objectives for the session: (1) helping members move toward their values by way of short-, medium-, and long-term goals, and (2) identifying some of the common barriers to committed action and how members can move through them. Let's examine these objectives more closely.

1. Developing goals that lead to valued living: The therapist wants to help all of her group members develop discrete, attainable goals in the service of their values. She would like them to experience success (defined as completing the committed action, not as a reward for doing so). Her hope is that by linking success to the choice to move, that action (a committed action in the service of values) will become intrinsically rewarding in and of itself. By delineating short-, medium-, and long-term goals, she helps members put shape to a path that takes them in the direction of their values.

2. Identifying barriers to committed action: The therapist will use a group exercise to illuminate some of the common barriers that can stand in the way of committed action. She also knows that as her members commit and begin to move, barriers will arise. She will use these opportunities to help the group members apply what they have learned in the therapy to respond to such barriers in a psychologically flexible way.

Developing Goals that Move Members Toward Their Values

We join our group after it has completed the Setting Your Intentions mindfulness exercise. The therapist works with the group members on any remaining questions they have around values and helps one or two refine theirs a bit. Aware of time, she moves immediately into the My Commitment exercise, which helps members identify value-driven actions while capitalizing on the group setting.

My Commitment
(developing and assisting committed action)

A group member writes "My _____ Commitment" along the top of the whiteboard and then names a commitment he or she is willing to work toward ("quit smoking," for example). The group then helps the member connect this commitment to a particular value and write that on the board (e.g., "In service of my value of being a loving father, I will quit smoking"). Next, the therapist has the group member write the column headings "Short Term," "Medium Term," and "Long Term" underneath the commitment described above.

The group then works with the group member to arrive at actions he is willing to do in order to move toward the stated value, placing them in the appropriate column.

The therapist, using the My Committed Action Worksheet, which includes the above-mentioned columns, writes down the committed actions generated by the members during the exercise (she will give the filled-out worksheet to each group member so that each has a record of what was developed).

Below is an illustration of these steps in action:

Therapist: Okay, group. Barry's made a commitment to go to the gym in the service of his health. Let's work together to see if we can't put some shape to that. Any ideas? (*Members think.*)

Mary: What if he packs a bag with his gym clothes in it, and puts it in his car?

Barry: That's actually a good idea! Might push me over that edge, you know?

Therapist: That *is* a great idea! Barry, when are you willing to do that?

Barry: I can do that tonight when I get home! (*applause from the group*)

Therapist: Great! Put that one under "short term."

The exercise continues until Barry has quite a number of items under each heading and the board looks like this:

My Committed Action Worksheet
My Gym Commitment

In service of my value of health, I commit to the following activities.

Short Term	Medium Term	Long Term
Put gym clothes in car.	Increase the number of times I go to the gym to twice per week.	Increase the number of times I go to the gym to 3–4 times a week.
Join the gym.	Find some workout buddies.	Join an organized class or team.
Go to the gym once.	Discover what types of exercise I really love.	

If she had more time, the therapist would have each member go to the board. However, she wants to put barriers to committed action explicitly on the table today so that group members might be enabled to recognize them should they arise before the next session. She asks for one more volunteer and has that member go to the whiteboard and follow the same procedure as Barry. Following this, she asks the group whether the exercise is clear and whether anyone has any questions (*members indicate they understand the task*). She then hands out blank My Committed Action Worksheets (see http://www.newharbinger.com/23994) and asks the remaining group members to take a few minutes to fill these out. (She asks the members who went to the whiteboard to do the same—she wants them to have a record of the goals they had identified). As members complete the handouts, the therapist observes and assists as needed. After about fifteen minutes, each member has arrived at a committed action and some specific goals.

The therapist has been reflecting on Barry's goals; she is a little suspicious of Barry's reaction during the whiteboard exercise. That is, he stated that he's been wanting to go to the gym for some time now, and she doubts that whatever was stopping him has gone away. His unbridled enthusiasm has her wondering whether Barry thinks he's been fixed now... She decides to go with this hypothesis as a means to explore barriers with the entire group.

Therapist:	Barry, you seem really excited about this. It's clear that reclaiming your health is important to you. I'm wondering what has kept you from doing this before. (*looks at him inquiringly*)
Barry:	Yeah, you're right. It's been pretty frustrating. I *wanted* to get to the gym. I just couldn't find the motivation to get going, no matter how much I know how good it would be for me.
Therapist:	What's different now?
Barry:	I feel psyched! I really want to get in there.
Therapist:	And have you felt that way before? Psyched to go?
Barry:	Yeah, I used to always feel that way. But then, I dunno—I just haven't felt motivated.
Therapist:	So feeling psyched was there, and then it wasn't. How long have you been waiting for motivation to show up?
Barry:	Well, a couple of years now.
Therapist:	What if you went to the gym without waiting for motivation to show up?
Barry:	(*a little taken aback*) Huh?
Therapist:	What if "feeling psyched" or "feeling motivated" were experiences to notice rather than something to wait for? What if you went to the gym right along with the feeling of un-motivation? What if you went tomorrow, even if you were no longer feeling psyched?
Barry:	(*slowly*) Okay…yeah, I could go regardless.
Therapist:	(*noncommittal*) Hmmm. *Or* you could wait some more for motivation, or maybe you could go only when you are feeling psyched—
Barry:	No. That's what I've been doing. (*is silent, considering*) No. I've waited long enough.
Therapist:	(*earnestly*) I look forward to hearing how this week goes for you, Barry, for all of you. Whatever has stopped you from living the way you want to be living is probably going to show up. You might feel psyched about making these moves, you might not. But this is about *choosing to move despite*, or *along with*, whatever's showing up. It's about moving toward what you have decided to care about in your lives.

The therapist spends the remainder of the session talking with the group about potential barriers, drawing upon their own experiences and helping them understand that committed action is not about *feeling* a certain way (e.g., motivated, certain, comfortable). Rather, it's about *holding* whatever is coming up around it and *moving* in a chosen direction.

Time is up for session 11 and the therapist needs to conclude the session. She has covered the main points she wanted members to grasp at an intellectual level regarding committed action—now it's time to swing into action. As much as she wants her members to get a taste of what it's like to live according to one's values, she wants them to recognize (even experience) the barriers that can arise so that she can work with these during the next and last session.

> *Therapist:* Okay. So all of you have identified one committed action you can take during the next week. Let's just go quickly around again and have each one of you state your commitment. (*Members state their commitments.*) Great. Wait, I need to state one too. (*thinks*) "In the service of my value of being a supportive friend, I commit to sending a card to a friend of mine who's having a tough time at work right now." Okay guys, let's do this! Please be your own observers during the week. See how aware you can be around this commitment—the thoughts that show up, the feelings, what you are doing or not doing, okay? (*Members assent.*) Great, I'll see you all next week!

We have come to session 12, the group's last therapy session, and our therapist is aware there's a lot to do. She wants to work with the group on the committed actions they declared in last week's session, really pulling in all of the core processes. That is, she wants to show how applying these abilities enables committed action, and how fusion, avoidance, and attachment to rules and self-concepts will also always be there as an available choice. She wants her group to recognize that such phenomena can always be noticed, and can always be accepted, while one is *doing* what works. She wants her group to connect again with self-as-context, that constant, inviolable awareness that is always there, larger than, and intact. Finally, she wants to express her appreciation for her group and their work together.

Session Strategy. The therapist will open session 12 with a brief mindfulness exercise called My Committed Action that points to committed action, while also directing attention to the Observing Self, the Noticer. She wants to reconnect her members to experiencing self-as-context before focusing on committed action. Her main objective for the session is to continue to tie the core processes together; she wants all group members to understand how psychological flexibility applies directly to their lives. She will lead a discussion about the committed actions declared last week, exploring and working through any barriers members experienced since last session. She wants to leave plenty of time for an experiential exercise (My Shrinking Life Space; M. Schmitz, personal communication, 2012) that reflects both the struggle members have been in and the opportunity before them now. She will conclude the therapy by sharing her appreciation for the group and allowing members to share whatever they would like to.

Tying the Processes Together

The therapist completes the brief mindfulness exercise, My Committed Action (emphasizing noticing the Noticer; see Supplemental Exercises at http://www.newharbinger.com/23994), and moves directly to a discussion about how members did with their committed actions. She has a good grasp of the common snares that can arise, and she listens for them as her group members talk about their experiences.

Therapist:	How about you Gina, how did it go? You picked a pretty challenging committed action last week as I recall. You were going to tell your mom you weren't coming to your sister's birthday party?
Gina:	(*looking troubled*) Yeah. I did it but—
Therapist:	You did it?! Fantastic! [*Although the therapist noticed the "but," she wants to first reinforce that Gina moved forward with her committed action.*]
Gina:	Yeah, but I felt *horrible* afterwards. She did the usual guilt trip thing. Now I'm wondering if I did the right thing.
Therapist:	(*leaning in*) Gina, this is it. You are so on it! You were really clear last week that in the service of self-care, you were choosing not to go home for that right now. You also had a pretty clear idea of the sorts of thoughts and feelings that would show up, and look: you chose, and they showed up. You have feelings of guilt, thoughts about having done the wrong thing, all that.
Gina:	You're probably going to say that I shouldn't buy my thoughts.
Therapist:	(*gently but very seriously*) I am 100% serious when I say that you get to buy them or not buy them. This is *your* life after all. And either way you choose, if you go ahead and go, or if you stay, there are going to be consequences—pros and cons. Only you can make the call of what you are, or are not, willing to experience. (*Gina is very quiet, thinking. The group is silent but listening intently.*)

Gina:	(*slowly*) No…I think I made the right choice. For me that is. I'm sure I'll feel guilty about it, though, but whatever.
Therapist:	(*turns her attention to the group. She is really leaning in, but at the same time trying not to convey that now Gina has made the "right" choice according to her—a tricky but important line to walk*) And here we have it folks. In making that choice, Gina is being *willing* to have the thoughts and feelings that come along. She is aware of them [willingness, contacting the present], noticing the thoughts that are coming up but not buying them [defusion, self-as-context], and making a choice that takes her closer to her values [values and committed action].
Therapist):	(*pausing to let this sink in; Gina looks very pleased with herself*) One thing to really watch for is the idea that if we make a strong move toward our values, we're going to be rewarded in some way, or that discomfort won't show up since we've made the "right" move, or that if discomfort *does* show up, we've made the "wrong" move. Feelings are going to come and go…the mind is going to do its thing; meanwhile, you are living in a way that is in line with how you want to show up in the world.

The therapist recognizes this is the perfect time to pull in the Passengers on the Bus metaphor (adapted from "Passengers on the Bus"; Hayes et al., 2011), and she does it now (see Supplemental Exercises at http://www.newharbinger.com/23994 for a description). Afterward, she has a strong impression that this metaphor was highly effective for the entire group. Her group members are nodding—the feel in the room is a bit electric—and her sense is that the full import of ACT has landed. She will now pull in an experiential exercise as a final punctuation mark to the work.

The therapist has come prepared with the My Shrinking Life Space handout (available at http://www.newharbinger.com/23994), writing tools, and tape, which she distributes to her group. She then proceeds as follows:

My Shrinking Life Space

(Schmitz, personal communication, 2012; committed action)

The therapist instructs the group to complete each section of the handout, offering examples to help them get started (e.g., write down something meaningful, something purposeful, something you used to do, something that you no longer engage in). She clarifies that these are things they used to do, or always wanted to do, but have been stopped by their thoughts, and she provides examples such as "I used to spend time with my friends" and "I always wanted to learn the guitar." (Note: Because the exercise is more illustrative when depicting aspects of group members' lives that were once there but are now lost, we suggest you save "something you have always wanted to do" for when people are stumped. This can happen with young people who haven't experienced these sorts of losses yet.)

Next, the therapist asks members to tear off the first thing they stopped doing and talk about it. (She cues them to limit this to a sentence or two in the interest of time.) She provides this example: "I used to play guitar, but after I got cut from an audition, I didn't think I was good enough to play anymore. I haven't picked it up since." (If you are doing this exercise with plenty of time, it is powerful to drop into this experience of loss a bit. With the guitar situation, for instance, you could have the group member contact what he felt in that moment long ago and what it has been like for him to notice the unopened guitar case.)

Once everyone has had a turn, she asks the group to silently tear off anything else that is no longer a part of their lives, and to leave the pieces that are still a part of their lives. (Some people might have one or two items still hanging on to the paper afterward, some might have none—all is fine.) The therapist invites them to fully contact what they experience as they tear it off of the paper. Because this can bring up powerful emotions, the therapist is careful to allow for plenty of time and space for whatever is showing up in the room. The therapist then instructs the group members to hold up their paper and discuss what it feels like to look at it.

Next, the therapist asks the members to pick up a piece and to identify what short-term goals they are willing to carry out in order to begin to put that piece back into their lives. She asks them to write that goal on the back of the piece and then tape it back onto the page. She has them tape it on backward, with the short-term goal facing front. For example, Dan, who wants to spend more time with his daughters, might write, "I will call my ex-wife and set up a father-daughter date." He would then tape the piece back on with the goal facing front. The therapist will encourage group members to help each other identify goals, but will stress that it is okay to leave a piece off if someone is not willing to work on it right now.

The therapist has everyone hold up their sheet with the pieces taped back on. She asks the group to describe what their life space looks like now. Because time allows, the therapist asks group members to share one or all of their committed action plans to bring the pieces back into their lives. She has each group member identify *one thing* he is willing to do *today* to put a piece back into his life. Finally, she has each group member stand up and state, "In service of my _____ value, I am willing to _____."

The therapist encourages the group members to keep their page nearby, even on the refrigerator if possible, as a tangible representation of a valued life.

Clinical Considerations in Working with Committed Action

Process over Content: Content is important here. It is essential to listen and discover what your group members are willing to commit to, always with an ear to common pitfalls to success. We don't forget to be aware of nonverbal cues and to always consider how things are actually functioning. If we see a group member cringe while committing, for example, we will go after that. Ultimately, committed action is all about process over content; members are guided to *move* despite whatever content shows up for them along the way.

Timing: Group members vary in terms of where they are with the core processes. At this point in the therapy that disparity can become particularly clear. That is, some group members might be energized and ready to get moving in their lives, while others are suddenly paralyzed at the thought of engaging in life again! As is so often the case, the group setting is invaluable in working with these differences. Stuck individuals learn from their peers who model moving forward despite discomfort. Those demonstrating more psychological flexibility in the moment learn from their peers who are stuck—inevitably even the most skillful member will encounter moments when thoughts are particularly sticky, when old behaviors emerge. We take care to notice what is happening in the room and use every opportunity to tie the core processes to what group members are experiencing.

Explicit versus nonexplicit intervention: Over the course of the therapy, values will appear. They will show up in what members say and do; they will be apparent in what causes them pain and in what brings them joy. We take such opportunities to gently point out that values are there (e.g., "It looks like you care about being a good mom"), knowing we will delve into this domain at a later point in the therapy. We also work with values nonexplicitly by helping the group connect with the pain of not living according to one's values. When we move explicitly to this core process, we put valued living squarely on the table, providing psychoeducation about how values and goals are viewed in ACT and helping members put their own values into words.

Experiential versus didactic work: We observed how our therapist used psychoeducation to help her group members develop committed actions in the service of their values, and actively tied concepts together. She used dialogue and examples to help her group understand how these abilities pertain to each of their lives, and most importantly, what valued living might bring. This demonstrates how we intentionally use the power of language in ACT to link values to actions, enhancing this by having group members articulate—both out loud and on paper—how they intend to show up in their lives.

Once again, we optimize experiential learning, making sure that group members have an opportunity to feel what putting these abilities into practice can bring. It is important to help members connect both with the suffering of a life that has become small, and with the qualities of a life imbued with meaning—*their* meaning.

Psychological flexibility is a matter of ongoing practice. The world will continue to present barriers, the mind will continue to present reasons and justifications for remaining stuck, and feelings will continue to be ungoverned. Holding these things differently will require practice. And yet, our therapist has given her group the skills to begin. Members have had a taste of living in a way that is vital and engaged. They have contacted the Self that is larger, experienced themselves as whole, and tasted the freedom that comes from letting internal experiences be while heading in a direction that matters.

Wrapping up this final session, our therapist finds herself very moved as she gazes at her group members, filled with gratitude for the way they have shown up for this therapy. Walking the walk, she shares her experience with the group, then she invites members to express whatever they would like to share. When they are done, there is a lot of emotion in the room. The group sits silently and savors the moment.

Summary

When their choices are in the service of values, group members have a road map to creating a life of purpose. In this chapter our therapist built this ability with her group, helping members understand how committed action brings all they learned in the therapy to the fore. She helped them put shape to a value-driven life and learn how to anticipate, recognize, and ultimately move through the barriers that can stand in the way. She provided opportunities to practice and use these skills to solidify the core processes, preparing her group for what lies ahead. Finally, she honored the work done by this group, sharing her experience and providing an opportunity for her group members to do the same.

We have completed the applied portion of this book, having worked through the core processes that help group members approach life in a way that is open, centered, and engaged. We have included some of the most common exercises and metaphors, mainly because they are effective ways to further the therapy in a group setting. We also made this choice because this is largely an introductory level text, and we wanted readers new to ACT to be familiar with exercises and metaphors that have become part of the vernacular (e.g., the Lemon, Lemon exercise, the man-in-a-hole metaphor, the Observer You exercise). However, for those of you who are experienced in ACT, we hope you have gained some additional exercises to add to your repertoire. Fortunately, there are many exercises and metaphors that can be used to create a powerful effect in a group setting. We point interested readers to the Supplemental Exercises available at http://www.newharbinger.com/23994, a compilation of excellent ACT group exercises both old and new.

CHAPTER 11

Conducting ACT in Different Types of Groups

One of the challenges in writing this book was deciding upon the parameters for the demonstration group depicted in chapters 4 through 10. ACT has been effectively implemented with all sorts of populations and settings (e.g., psychiatric wards, long- and short-term treatment programs, outpatient groups) and in all sorts of ways—from an immersive, several-hours-a-week treatment to a single-session intervention. In fact, one of the strengths of the ACT model is that it lends itself well to this sort of tailoring.

This makes sense when we remember that ACT is a principle-based treatment. Developing psychological flexibility via the six core processes is not dependent upon particular content; it does not require a particular order or technique. The interrelatedness of the processes further enhances flexibility. Group facilitators can target what they feel would be best for their group, knowing they are not so much choosing one process at the cost of another, but rather homing in on a skill they deem particularly important for their group members (and that other interrelated abilities likely will be furthered as part of this endeavor).

We elected to demonstrate the therapy as it might unfold in a weekly, outpatient, closed-group setting wherein the therapist is working through the core ACT processes in a sequential fashion. We felt this provided the best opportunity to fully explore each process, to demonstrate how each might manifest in session and how members are guided to increase their abilities with all six.

It is easy to misconstrue such an approach as being rigid or content driven, and we have taken pains to show otherwise. For example, we showed how this approach is not necessarily linear and how the therapist might linger on one core process or revisit those previously introduced depending upon what is happening in her group. We also showed how the therapist can recognize and effectively work with whatever processes naturally arise in the therapy, regardless of where one is in terms of sequence. We explained that the sequential approach is more about what is explicitly pointed out in session than about what processes are actually being worked on. That is, there are many ways to further members' abilities with all the processes even while selecting one process as the topic of the session, and we provided numerous examples of how this can be done.

Our hope in taking this approach was that once readers had an understanding of the processes and how to recognize and work with them within the dynamics of a group, they would gain a sense of how this might translate to other sorts of groups. To further this translation, we will use this chapter to demonstrate some of the different ways ACT can be implemented. We have selected examples that reflect some of the most significant differences in group type: (1) an open-ended, drop-in group (where members are coming and going); (2) a brief inpatient group that meets for only four sessions; (3) an open-ended, sequential format; and (4) a single-session group intervention. In exploring these scenarios, we'll discuss the key considerations that come into play and how these influence the work. Finally, we will address some of the challenges of each approach and offer tips as to how to work with them.

Example Group 1: Open-Ended, Drop-In Group

The first type of group we'll explore is one in which membership is open and attendance is variable. In a moment we'll discuss the specific parameters of our example group and their implications, but first, we'll touch on more general considerations that arise when we conduct this type of ACT group.

Clinical Considerations for an Open-Ended, Drop-In Group

Group cohesion/support: While time-limited, closed-membership groups might more easily bond, structuring the group so that individuals can come and go does not rule out a supportive group culture. In fact, by working within the ACT model, the therapist can build a powerful group zeitgeist that moves with the group as a whole even as membership varies from session to session. With consistent modeling and reinforcing of skills such as contacting the present, willingness, and committed action, for example, a growth-enhancing culture is established that shapes the behavior of whoever is attending the group. In our sample session below we will demonstrate how this can be done.

Choosing what to focus on and tying things together: This is arguably the most challenging clinical consideration when conducting ACT with this type of group. With attendance and membership fluctuating, we can't rely on multiple sessions to get ideas across or to pull things together. How do we get enough ACT done in each session to be helpful to those who are there? We are assisted by remembering the pragmatic goal of ACT—to get members unstuck and moving forward in their lives. If we consider what this means for the particular members of a group, it becomes clear where to focus in session. Additionally, in emphasizing this "moving with your feet" objective of ACT, we can get down to meaningful work quickly. As we will see in the example below, moving with one's feet requires all of the core processes. We will be able to quickly see where members are stuck and will have ample opportunities to develop the skills they need to get unstuck.

Introducing processes in an accessible, immediately applicable way: In any given group, there could be individuals attending for the first time alongside those who have participated every week for months. You could have one member who is well versed in the difference between looking *at* versus *from* thoughts, for instance, and another brand new member who has no experience with it at all. This means that throughout the group, it will be particularly important to use language that is easy to understand and to have several exercises on hand that provide straightforward illustrations of key concepts. Working with examples that occur in the moment will be key.

We cannot stress enough that the ACT model works well here. All the processes will be in play in every session, providing the therapist with ample opportunity to point to whatever she deems helpful in that session. Also, there is no point of mastery, which means that even if a member has heard about and practiced defusion a dozen times, he can still benefit from ongoing practice and application of this skill in his daily life.

Keeping things fresh: As therapists become more facile with ACT, they often find themselves creating novel exercises on the fly or running with metaphors that group members introduce. And of course, therapists can draw upon a wealth of exercises and metaphors to keep things interesting. However, it's worth noticing the tendency to feel pressure to be "fresh" in the first place. In other words, the life in this group will come from the in-the-moment connection between and among the therapist and participants. As members interact and share their thoughts, feelings, and day-to-day experiences, there will be plenty of opportunities to infuse vitality and meaning into the session.

Keeping momentum going: When group members have attended meetings over a long period of time, it is important to keep forward movement front and center. It is easy for these members to rest on their laurels and become "junior therapists" as a way of avoiding their own work. Keep track of their verbal commitments and watch for the person staying stuck.

Parameters of Example Group 1

Our open-membership example group is an outpatient, self-referred (voluntary) drop-in group for individuals struggling with addiction. The group meets twice weekly for fifty minutes. Let's take a moment to examine the variables just mentioned:

Outpatient setting: There are many possible explanations as to why a given group member is seeking outpatient treatment as opposed to more intensive treatment alternatives. Pragmatically speaking, group members are apparently functioning well enough that hospitalization isn't in order. It is also likely that group members are spending a lot of time in contexts that run counter to the ideas purported in ACT. This can especially be the case when working with addiction, so additional support (e.g., individual therapy, supplemental ACT texts and handouts, readings, Alcoholics Anonymous meetings) and between-session tasks that keep ACT processes at the forefront could be helpful.

Self-referred: An implication here is that group members recognize that they are in trouble and need assistance. This is "therapeutic gold" and can be used to pull members forward into lives that they find valuable and vital. There will likely be opportunities to use this move—seeking treatment—as an example of psychological flexibility. That is, although members have thoughts and feelings to the contrary, they nonetheless show up for group (demonstrating willingness, defusion, values, and committed action).

Drop-in: The fact that members come and go means that each session needs to offer something in their endeavor to remain sober. The therapist will not have the luxury of gradually building a case here, but will need to get to the heart of the matter in every session (we will demonstrate this shortly). Selecting experiential exercises and metaphors that nicely reflect all or most of the core processes will be key.

Twice weekly for fifty minutes: As said, there is no way to know for sure when and how often individuals will attend this group. Because it meets twice weekly, it is possible that some members will attend quite frequently while others may come rarely. The therapist can draw upon regularly attending members to help new or less frequently attending members progress. He will also be able to refer back to previous discussions in a way that reinforces key ideas for some members and introduces them to others.

Fifty minutes is not a lot of time, especially if there are several group members in attendance. It will be easy to stray off course. Structuring the session a bit to set the stage for ACT will help.

Population of individuals with addiction: Although the core processes are applicable to human beings in general, the manner in which ACT is delivered is certainly influenced by group membership. Which exercises and metaphors to use, what words to use, whether and how deeply to explore a topic…all are considered in light of who's in the group and the goals for the therapy.

If we consider these choices in terms of this group, the ACT processes of defusion, willingness, and committed action stand out. That is, central to members' progress will be the ability to notice but not buy in to thoughts and feelings about using/drinking, that is, to notice and simply hold urges and discomfort while choosing to remain sober. This guides the therapist to create and look for opportunities in every session to build these skills.

The therapist will also seek opportunities to help members contact deeply held values. Clearly, something is pulling them to group. Clarifying their values—how they would like to show up in the world—will be vital work.

Sample Group 1 Session

We will describe one hypothetical session to demonstrate what ACT might look like in a group of this sort. In this sample session our therapist will open the group with a mindfulness exercise. He has found that contacting the present tends to be very difficult for individuals struggling with addiction, and he wants to provide an opportunity for practice. Starting with a mindfulness exercise also sets the stage for the work, marking the group as an ACT session and providing some structure.

As for the rest of the session, the therapist intentionally leaves it fairly open-ended. He wants to make room for what members bring to session, but he'll be viewing everything that unfolds though an ACT lens. He will continually be seeking opportunities to pull out core ACT processes, helping members recognize deficits (e.g., avoidance in the place of willingness, fusion in the place of just noticing thoughts) and providing opportunities to build their abilities.

This is not to say the therapist has no agenda. Simply put, it is to help members stay sober and move forward in their lives. Every core ACT process is reflected in that fundamental goal. By keeping this objective front and center, the therapist knows the group will be working actively with what has been keeping members stuck, and developing the skills needed to get unstuck.

Finally, the therapist is armed with several ACT metaphors and exercises that he thinks will be particularly effective for this group and that, given its open nature, will nicely reflect all the core processes. In particular, because defusion and willingness play such a pivotal role in maintaining sobriety, he comes prepared with experiential exercises that will help members build those skills. He will be drawing upon these to tie important ACT concepts and skills together (see the Supplemental Exercises at http://www.newharbinger.com/23994 for a collection of such exercises, along with those described in chapters 5 through 10).

We join the group as members take their seats in order to begin the session:

Therapist: Welcome everybody!

(Members greet the therapist and one another as they settle in their seats.)

Therapist: *(noticing a new group member)* Hi, I'm Tom. You're new to this group.

New group member:	Yeah, I'm Mike.
Therapist:	Hi Mike, and welcome. (*Therapist looks around, sees an individual who has not been to the group in some time*). Hey, Jake! Good to see you!
Jake:	(*looking a little sheepish*) Hey. Yeah…it's been a little rough lately.
Therapist:	(*smiling and nodding understandingly*) Then I'm all the gladder you made the choice to be here! I want to hear more about what helped you do that. But first let's all spend a few moments getting centered. Let's do a quick mindfulness exercise to get present.

Notice that the therapist's response to Jake's "it's been a little rough" focused on process rather than content. That is, rather than asking why things had been rough, the therapist focused on the fact that Jake made a behavioral choice—a committed action—which he then quickly moved to verbally reinforce (i.e., "I'm all the gladder…"). Jake's demeanor led him to hypothesize that Jake was experiencing some shame, and rather than attempt to assuage that, his response (including his warm nonverbal behavior) aimed to (a) emphasize what is within Jake's control (whether or not to come) and (b) undermine what Jake's mind was likely handing him (e.g., that the therapist would judge him, be disappointed in him).

Therapist:	(*to new member*) Mike, are you familiar at all with mindfulness?
Mike:	Um, I'm not sure…not really.
Therapist:	(*to the group*) Who can tell Mike what mindfulness is *not*?
Group member:	It is not about contemplating your navel (group laughs).
Therapist:	(*laughing along*) Ok, that's true. (*to Mike*) It's not about navel gazing or about trying to relax, or really trying to be anything. We are working on just noticing what is happening at any given moment, thoughts, feelings, sensations in your body. We tend to get up in our heads and this is a way to get back in touch with our lives.

In this example the therapist is only going to spend about three to five minutes guiding the group in a mindfulness exercise. He'll simply guide members to notice the sounds in the room, their breathing, and that they have thoughts and feelings that are showing up as they do the exercise. He doesn't want to lose the interest of the new member before he's even gotten going, and he knows that simply sitting in this way can be a real challenge for individuals struggling with addiction. If he had come into the group and noticed that everyone there was a regular attendee, he might have elected to do a longer mindfulness exercise.

> *Therapist:* (*having concluded the mindfulness exercise*) So, maybe we can start with what you shared, Jake—that things have been rough for you lately. What have you been experiencing? [*This word choice is deliberate—the therapist is pulling for defusion, self-as-process and self-as-context here.*]

> *Jake:* (*hesitantly*) Well…I had a slip. (*stops, looks around the group to see members' reactions. Therapist nods very compassionately and understandingly at Jake, says nothing. Jake waits for more reaction, but the group follows the therapist's lead and sits silently.*)

> *Jake:* So that's it. (*sits back in his chair, signaling he is very ready to move on to something else*)

At this point our therapist chooses to sit silently for a few moments. He hypothesizes that Jake is attempting to move off of discomfort, and he takes the opportunity to develop willingness in the place of avoidance. That is, he does not want Jake's behavior to function as avoidance, so rather than taking the cue to move on, the therapist instead models simply having the experience, and then creates an opportunity for Jake to do the same:

> *Therapist:* I'm wondering what it's like for you to say that, Jake. What are you experiencing right in this moment?

> *Jake:* I'm embarrassed! I'm pissed at myself. (*falls silent, therapist and group just sit silently with him*)

> *Jake:* (*suddenly moving restlessly in his chair*) I don't know. I shouldn't even be here! (*looks at the clock*)

> *Therapist:* Yeah, it looks like you want to fly right out of that chair! (*Jake is silent.*)

Here the therapist is noting Jake's discomfort and apparent desire to leave the room (avoidance). He is noticing Jake is fused with his thoughts and hypothesizes that his restlessness, clock-watching, and even his anger function to stave off other uncomfortable feelings (suggesting a lack of willingness, contacting the present, defusion).

> *Therapist:* I really appreciate your honesty Jake…it isn't easy to share what you did, but you stepped in. [*The therapist could focus on the avoidance, but chooses to reinforce the willingness and committed action Jake also demonstrated.*]

Therapist:	(*to group*) We've talked about willingness in here…can anyone share with Mike what we mean by willingness?
Group member:	Willingness is when you just have whatever it is you're experiencing. You know, bad thoughts or feelings. You don't try to escape them.
Therapist:	That's right, whether it's an urge to drink, or a tough thought or just feeling antsy. But that isn't always easy, is it? (*Members nod in agreement.*) Even now, there's all sorts of stuff happening in here. So Jake demonstrated willingness by coming and sharing today even though he wasn't happy about having had a slip, even though he had all sorts of thoughts about what would happen in here. (*to Jake*) Is that safe to say Jake? (*Jake nods*). We all are experiencing stuff right now. (*pauses, modeling contacting the present*) I notice myself feeling glad that Jake's here… I have lots of thoughts going on too… (*to group*) What are some of the things you guys are noticing?
Group member:	I feel real tense.
Group member:	I just totally get where Jake's coming from. I mean, we've all had relapses and it's not fun.
Therapist:	(*staying on point and in the moment with the core processes*) Well, and we've had plenty of times in here where tough stuff comes up, just like right now. And notice how we can just notice and hold it. (*to Mike*) This is what we mean by willingness. All sorts of thoughts, feelings, even physical sensations come up, AND, we don't actually have to fix them or escape them or drink them away…we can choose to be willing to just hold them. (*sits silently with the group for a bit*)
Therapist:	Jake, I'm wondering what helped you choose to come today. Do you remember what you were experiencing as you made that decision?
Jake:	(*looking a bit more settled*) I just knew I needed to come. That if I didn't I might use again.
Therapist:	Wow. Can you tell us again why it's so important to you not to drink?
Jake:	I want my life back! I want to be able to be a good dad to my kids…to keep my job…I can't do any of it if I go back to drinking.
Therapist:	So you have a value around what kind of dad you are, values around working—

Jake: You bet.

Therapist: And you chose to pursue those values by coming in today, even though you had thoughts and feelings about it.

Jake: Yeah. I *really* didn't want to tell the group I'd slipped. But…it's not so bad.

Therapist: Yeah, even though your mind told you all sorts of things about today, here you are!

At this point the therapist feels key processes have been highlighted (e.g., willingness, defusion, values, committed action) and he wants to turn his attention to other members of the group. Pulling in an exercise or metaphor that punctuates the processes that are in play would work nicely at this point. Passengers on the Bus would be compelling, for example, with Jake depicted as driving the bus toward sobriety despite attempted interference by some unruly passengers (e.g., relapse, embarrassment, fear of judgment; see Supplemental Exercises at http://www.newharbinger.com/23994 for a detailed description of this metaphor and how it also can be done as an experiential exercise). This is a way to introduce the new group member to a powerful ACT metaphor while also benefitting the more seasoned members. We have never found it problematic to judiciously revisit previously introduced metaphors—in fact, when we apply familiar metaphors to new situations, the applicability of the processes becomes even more clear.

As the session draws to a close, the therapist asks group members to take a few moments to consider what they are hoping to accomplish by coming to this group. After allowing them time to contact this, he asks them to consider a move they could take that is in support of remaining sober. He asks a seasoned group member to provide an example:

Therapist: Glen, are you willing to share what came up for you? What move are you willing to make this week that's in line with your intention to remain sober?

Glen: I'm going to come to this group on Thursday. Also going to pass on a birthday party I've been invited to—it'll be just one big party.

Therapist: Great. Anyone else care to share before we wrap up? (*Several members share.*)

Therapist: (*ending the session*) Okay, thanks everybody. Mike, thanks for being a part of this group today.

In this example we saw how ACT can be done in a group with varying membership. In essence, each session must stand alone. By remaining focused on the core ACT processes, the therapist was able to highlight and help his group develop the abilities needed to remain sober within the confines of one fifty-minute session. There is an important difference between this example and ACT as a single intervention, however. That is, although in both cases each session needs to have enough ACT substance to be constructive, the continuing nature of an open-ended group plays a large role in the treatment. Throughout this session the therapist drew upon the fact that the group has been ongoing (e. g., soliciting helpful input from more seasoned members). One gets the sense that he has managed to establish a group culture that now facilitates the work in each session.

Example Group 2: Limited-Session Group

There are many reasons why a therapist might have only a few group sessions to deliver ACT. Frequently, the therapist is targeting a particular clinical issue, for example, chronic pain, anger, depression…the list goes on. (See the Association for Contextual Behavioral Science [ACBS] website at http://www.contextualscience.org for several protocols.) As we have seen, the features of each particular group influence how ACT is delivered. For this example, we will use an outpatient, provider-referred group for individuals diagnosed with depression that meets for four ninety-minute sessions over two weeks. Our focus will be on some of the clinical considerations that pertain to this limited-session example.

Clinical Considerations for a Limited-Session Group

Population of individuals diagnosed with depression: That group members are referred by their providers suggests (but does not necessitate) a certain level of severity. That is, these individuals have sought treatment for depression, received a diagnosis, and were deemed in need of additional treatment. Their struggle with depressive symptoms points to deficits in certain ACT core processes. For example, we can anticipate that members will be highly fused with their minds and experientially avoidant. There may be significant deficits in self-as-process as well. That is, individuals struggling with depression often view themselves as *being* depressed—as though depression has landed on them and overtaken them, rather than viewing it as a constellation of thoughts, feelings, and sensations they are currently experiencing. Bringing an awareness to the ongoing flow of experience will be critical for this group (e.g., mindfulness exercises in each session; encouraging daily practice; tasking members to write down what they are thinking, feeling, and sensing in a given moment). It will also be beneficial to help them distinguish between these internal experiences and the Experiencer (self-as-context), and the treatment will incorporate experiential exercises such as the Label Parade (see Supplemental Exercises at http://www.newharbinger.com/23994), geared toward developing this ability.

Four, ninety-minute sessions: Because this group is going to meet for only four sessions, the therapy will need to be designed such that most of the core processes are pulled in right away. Active, experiential exercises such as the aforementioned Label Parade and Take Your Mind for a Walk (Hayes et al., 2011) work well here. (See Supplemental Exercises at http://www.newharbinger.com/23994 for instructions for this exercise.) The brevity of this group also augments the need for our therapist to assign between-session work designed to get members moving between sessions.

A drawback to a time-limited group, especially when compared with groups that meet more frequently, is that it can be harder to gain momentum. This is one of the reasons for designing tasks that will get members moving with their feet (committed action). As with longer treatment approaches, it will be important to draw a clear thread through the therapy—to link each session to the one before so that it will all come together.

The following group example demonstrates what this might look like rolled out in four sessions.

Sample Group 2 Sessions

In the first session, the therapist is tasked with establishing a culture that is supportive and also gets members moving—time is short! He gathers information regarding how group members perceive their situations and how "depression" (as they refer to it) is functioning in their lives. Using an approach similar to the creative hopelessness technique described in chapter 5, the therapist generates a discussion regarding what members have tried to do to "fix their depression" and, while careful to validate their suffering, brings the unworkability of that agenda to the fore. This takes up much of the session. To undermine avoidance, the therapist doesn't want to move too quickly to what's next (otherwise, group members could perceive whatever he presented as "the solution"). However, he is mindful of the time constraints and wants to get values on the table quickly as a way to pull the group forward into action. He asks the group, "If you weren't experiencing these depressed thoughts and feelings" (note the distinction being made between Experiencer and experiences), "what would you be doing? Do you have a vision for what your life would be if you weren't struggling with this stuff?"

During the ensuing discussion, the therapist helps his group identify values. He does so lightly; that is, he doesn't verbally wrestle with members in a way that forces ACT-consistent values (e.g., "Rather than pursing happiness—which doesn't work—what about being engaged in life?"). Rather, he points to values reflected in what the group is sharing:

Therapist: (to member who shared that if she wasn't depressed, she would have energy to do things with her kids and exercise more) If that experience of low energy wasn't standing in the way, you're saying you would engage with your kids more, take care of your physical health?

Group member: Yeah (suddenly tearful). I hate it when my kids see me this way.

Therapist: *(gently)* You really care about that, how you show up for your kids.

Group member: *(whispers)* Yes. Yes I do.

Therapist: That's really what we're about here. Helping you get back into lives that you value.

The therapist then introduces the Clarifying Values Worksheet (Walser & Westrup, 2007, see http://www.newharbinger.com/23994) and goes over it with the group. Again, he wants to emphasis that this (values) needs to come from them, and he describes the task as "an exploration to see what you care about in your heart of hearts." He asks each member to work with the sheets and bring them to the next session.

In session two, the therapist discusses the Clarifying Values Worksheet and spends a few minutes helping members with any questions or difficulties they encountered. (If members haven't finished with it, he asks them to continue to work on it between sessions.) He segues from this discussion to the topic of misapplied control (e.g., the fix-it agenda) by commenting that he is struck by the group's desire to engage in life, and that it may be that the experience of depression isn't what's holding them back. Again, careful to be compassionate and accepting of their experience, he suggests that control or avoidance may be what's standing in the way. He employs the Tug-of-War exercise (see chapter 5) to demonstrate both the suffering and futility of battling the experience of depression and to introduce willingness as viewed in ACT. He pulls in the values work by making the point that if members choose to drop the rope, they are free to move in the direction of their values.

Nearing the end of the second session, the therapist distributes Self-as-Context Tracking Sheets (Walser & Westrup, 2007; see http://www.newharbinger.com/23994) and asks the group members to "become detectives" when they experience depression. That is, he asks that two or three times between now and the next session, when noticing they are feeling depressed, they use the form to notice and record the ongoing flow of experience—to write down the thoughts they are having, the emotions that show up, and any physical sensations they can identify (self-as-process). He asks them to bring these self-as-context worksheets to the next session.

In the third session, the therapist aims to bring all the core processes into play. He begins the session with a mindfulness exercise to (a) provide an opportunity for the group to practice, and (b) tie in both willingness and the self-as-process work started with the detective homework (i.e., he guides them to notice the thoughts, feelings, and sensations that arise during the exercise and "hold them lightly like a butterfly"). He also guides them to "notice the Noticer" (*self-as-context*) and, following the exercise, discusses what is meant by the Noticer.

Next, the therapist talks explicitly about looking at, versus from, thoughts (defusion) using as examples some of the thoughts members noted in their detective work. He employs the Take Your Mind for a Walk exercise, pulling in the previous self-as-context work by referring to the person who

180

is being followed by the mind as "the Noticer." Finally, he introduces the Label Parade exercise (Walser & Westrup, 2007; see Supplemental Exercises at http://www.newharbinger.com/23994) to further develop self-as-context. Because only thirty minutes are left in the session, he conducts the exercise with just one group member. For homework, the group members refer to their Clarifying Values Worksheets and articulate one committed action they will take before the last group session.

The fourth and final session opens with a mindfulness meditation followed by a discussion of the committed actions declared at the end of the last session. As both successes and barriers are explored, the therapist will illuminate the processes of being present, willingness, defusion, self-as-context, values, and committed action. He draws a thread through the therapy by reviewing what the group has done over four sessions and also provides a list of resources to help them continue their ACT journey. He wraps up the session with the Passengers on the Bus Metaphor (see the Supplemental Exercises at http://www.newharbinger.com/23994.)

Example Group 3: Open-Membership, Sequential Group

ACT's very flexibility makes it challenging to categorize! For example, though we could purport that the sequential approach described in chapters 4 through 9 works best when groups have closed membership and are starting and ending the therapy together, we can also offer examples that contradict such a summation. In fact, in her intensive outpatient program (IOP) for anxiety, Joann has developed a group intervention that effectively delivers ACT in a sequential fashion even as new members can join the group at any point. We'll use this as our next example group, starting with a basic group description. We'll then explore some of the clinical implications of this iteration of an ACT group and provide a sample curriculum.

This IOP for anxiety takes place in a behavioral health hospital outpatient center. Members are referred to the program through the hospital's referral center or as a step-down process from either an inpatient program or a partial hospitalization program (PHP). Therefore, group members are admitted and discharged at any time, though most stay for an average of four weeks.

ACT is delivered as a group intervention (averaging eight to twelve members) Monday through Friday for three hours per day. The session frequency and length allows the therapist to move through the therapy in a sequential fashion, so although members might enter the group midweek or even on a Friday, they will receive at least one full course of ACT by the time they are discharged. Because the curriculum repeats every week, most patients will revisit (meaning they will participate in a session focused on) each core process several times during their enrollment in the program.

Clinical Considerations for an Open-Membership, Sequential Group

Let's take a look at the clinical considerations for this group:

Open membership: The behavioral health hospital must be able to admit patients at any time, so open, rolling admission to the IOP is necessary. This allows for treatment accessibility but incurs a particular challenge as well. That is, interventions either must be offered as stand-alone sessions or must tolerate changing group membership. At the same time, the typical length of stay creates ample opportunity to implement treatments that build skills day by day. Joann's team opted to take advantage of the latter approach and developed an ACT curriculum that focuses on a different core process each day, five days in a row, with one core process, contacting the present, infused into each session (as will be seen below).

To address the fact that any given group may consist of brand new members and those who have participated for weeks, a scaffolding technique is employed. "Scaffolding" refers to drawing upon more seasoned group members to assist in teaching the core processes and skills to the newer group members (similar to what occurred in the first example group). There are several advantages to this approach. The act of articulating and demonstrating the processes so that newer members can learn deepens the skills of those doing the teaching. The therapist is also provided information regarding members' understanding of what has been covered, and can clarify or reinforce as appropriate. New group members are encouraged and often inspired by the progress evident in the more seasoned group members.

To provide an example, Joann recalls a particular group member who eagerly took notes during her first ACT session (which was focusing on defusion). As the therapist began to explore defusion, the group member interrupted and asked (with pencil poised to write down a quick answer), "Okay, how do we do that?" The therapist hypothesized this member was experiencing discomfort around "not knowing" and took the opportunity to open this up for discussion with the group.

Therapist:	(*to new member*) Before we go there, do you mind if I have you check in for a moment? What are you feeling right now?
New member:	I dunno. Sort of lost to be honest.
Therapist:	(*nodding understandingly*) That's understandable! And is it safe to say you're asking a lot of questions and writing things down as a way to fix that? (*Group member nods.*)
Therapist:	(*speaking to the group*) Who here can relate? (*Members chuckle and raise their hands.*) Yeah, me too! Sometimes my mind goes absolutely bonkers when I feel confused or

like I don't know something. [*Although there are many productive directions in which to head with this, the therapist is turning the group's attention to thoughts to pave the way for the defusion focus of the session.*]

Therapist: (*speaking to group member who, being in his third week of the program, has attended two sessions focused on defusion*) David, can you provide some examples of what your mind might hand you when you're feeling confused or anxious?

After using what David shares as examples of what the mind can hand one when confused or anxious, the therapist could then ask David or another experienced group member to describe what is meant by fusion and defusion in ACT (or, if simpler wording is desired, the difference between buying in to thoughts and simply noticing thoughts). This scaffolding technique not only optimizes the rich learning opportunities in groups, but also provides the therapist a continuing opportunity to assess members' progress.

A potential drawback of implementing a sequential approach in this setting is the possibility that a group member may be prematurely discharged before receiving the full curriculum, which occurs on rare occasion. However, given the setting and population needs, Joann and her team felt the advantages of delivering ACT in this sequential manner outweighed that risk. They take care to mitigate the potential cost of an early discharge by providing referrals to a known ACT therapist in the area and recommending ACT self-help books focused on the individual's area of struggle.

Three-hour daily sessions: With this level of intensity, momentum is an advantage. New group members can be brought up to speed quickly, and those who have been in group longer can deepen their understanding of the core processes. The ample session length allows for a rich mix of psychoeducation, dialogue, and experiential work. Let's take a look at what the intervention looks like over the course of a week.

Weekly Agenda for Example Group 3

To develop the group curriculum, the therapists in this IOP plan out four weeks of sessions. We provide the schedule for week one below. The group therapists make sure that various exercises and metaphors are used each week to keep sessions fresh and to maximize different ways of working on the core processes.

There are a few things to notice about this agenda. One is that contacting the present is worked on each session via a mindfulness exercise. This is because contacting the present moment is not only a fundamental skill but is also hard to develop (particularly with individuals who have anxiety). In this intervention, group members will have an opportunity for daily practice.

Notice also that the therapist begins each session by reviewing the committed actions that members stated at the end of the previous session they were willing to do before the next session. (On Friday, group members are instructed to pick two: one for each weekend day.) Every session opens with all members discussing their committed action and whether or not they were able to accomplish their efforts. If so, they share with the group the successful experience, and if not, the barriers to success are explored. This discussion provides an opportunity to pull in previously learned processes (and for new members, to begin to develop familiarity).

The first half of the session is thus spent in review followed by a mindfulness exercise. Following a break, the second half focuses on exploring the core ACT process for the day. This schedule remains the same week after week, but as mentioned, the group leaders introduce new exercises for each process over four weeks.

MONDAY	TUESDAY	WEDNESDAY	THURSDAY	FRIDAY
Review of committed action from the weekend. Mindfulness exercise: Welcome Anxiety	Review of committed action from the night before. Mindfulness exercise: Tonglen	Review of committed action from the night before. Mindfulness exercise: "Don't Move!"	Review of committed action from the night before. Mindfulness exercise: Sensation Station	Review of committed action from the night before. Mindfulness exercise: Notice the Room for the First Time
Defusion exercise: Silly Voices	Acceptance exercise: Fall in Love	Self-as-context exercise: Eyes On	Values exercise: Finding Values in Life Experiences	Committed action exercise: Stand Up for Your Values
Wrap up: Committed action for tonight	Wrap up: Committed action for tonight	Wrap up: Committed action for tonight	Wrap up: Committed action for tonight	Wrap up: Committed actions for the weekend

The group intervention detailed in this example highlights the flexibility of the ACT model even when implemented in a fairly structured curriculum. The benefits of the therapy are potentiated while the particular needs of this treatment setting and population are met.

Example Group 4: Single-Session Intervention

In this exploration of different types of ACT groups, we would be remiss if we did not include a single-session example. It may seem far-fetched that ACT can effectively be conveyed in such a brief amount of time, but fortunately it can be done. In many settings, that is the only opportunity the provider will have (we refer interested readers to *Brief Interventions for Radical Change: Principles and Practice of Focused Acceptance and Commitment Therapy*, by Strosahl, Robinson, and Gustavsson [2012]).

Let's jump right into a working example. This will be a ninety-minute session for people who have recently had spinal cord surgery and are facing the prospect of living with chronic pain. This group meets in a hospital setting, before the patients are sent home following their surgery. The group therapist runs this group once per week.

Clinical Considerations for a Single-Session Intervention

Here are some of the factors that influence how ACT is delivered in this type of group:

Population of individuals with chronic pain: Living with chronic pain is a major challenge. Individuals are tasked with coming to terms with what they may experience as unacceptable—unrelenting pain. And yet, the choice is to either move forward and live one's life, or stop. We are immediately guided to core ACT processes that will be required for this monumental life: willingness and committed action in the service of one's values.

Possible first exposure to psychotherapy: Another aspect of this group worth mentioning is that these individuals are receiving this intervention as a standard follow up to their medical procedure. It is likely that many members will have no prior experience with psychotherapy. The language used in this intervention will need to be as clear and free of jargon as possible.

Single session: It may seem impossible to impart the essential aspects of the ACT model in a single ninety-minute session. However, we can return to the essential goal of ACT—to get members unstuck and moving forward in their lives—as a guide. The therapist will need a hook here, something that will pull the group forward despite the presence of pain. Identification and clarification of deeply held values will be key. The therapist also can anticipate barriers to valued living: the experience of pain and fusion with what the mind says about that experience. Developing willingness and learning how to defuse from thoughts will be particularly important for this group.

Session Strategy for Example Group 4

To aid in her endeavor, the therapist will introduce a worksheet, a revised version of the Mindful Action Plan, developed by D. J. Moran (2013). The Mindful Action Plan (available at http://www. newharbinger.com/23994) is a single-page worksheet that centers on the simple statement "I am here now, accepting the way I feel and noticing my thoughts, while doing what I care about." Notice how this encompasses all the core processes of ACT. Also included is a "to do" list (to reflect committed action), with sections for goal setting and accountability. She will incorporate this tool in her single-session agenda as shown below.

Note that although use of a tool such as the Mindful Action Plan can help distill ACT to a single-session intervention, the therapist must still have a solid grasp of the model. Just about anything can happen in a session like this, and looking consistently through that ACT lens and working with the core processes will guide the therapist to respond in a way that moves things forward.

Sample Group 4 Session

The therapist will begin the session by welcoming participants. As always, style is extremely important. That is, embodying and modeling the core processes will help create an environment conducive to growth. For example, it would be unwise for the therapist to attempt to cheerlead or otherwise fix what her group members are experiencing at this time in their lives. However, she can model willingness, values, and committed action right off the bat:

Therapist: Welcome everybody. (*long pause as she looks around at everyone in the group*) You know, I actually have a lot of mixed feelings going on. On the one hand, I am glad you've come because I believe you may find something helpful here. Something important. On the other hand, who am I to suggest there's a way to deal with what you're going through? (*members are listening attentively*) In fact, I think that's where we should start. I would really like to have a sense of what this is like for you. Is anyone willing to share what's going on for you right now?

The therapist is working to establish a supportive, authentic group culture as quickly as possible. She modeled defusion, self-as-process, values, and committed action with her opening statements, and she is now pulling for others to share their experience as well. (Notice that her word choice, "…to share what's going on for you," pulls for self-as-process). In the ensuing conversation, the therapist will pull for examples of fusion with thoughts, such as ruined expectations or dire predictions about a future with chronic pain. Throughout, she will continue to model willingness, validating her members' thoughts and feelings while also not attempting to fix what they are experiencing.

Therapist:	So now we have it. (*long pause*) Everything you've said makes perfect sense to me. I'm pretty sure that were I in your shoes, I would be feeling the same way. Soooo. (*looks at the group inquiringly*)
Group member 1:	So now what?
Therapist:	Yes, exactly! *That* is the question! (*Group members look at her silently, taking this in.*) You know, I hear so much caring in what you've shared. (*to one group member*) You clearly have so much grief around not being able to play baseball with your son anymore. There is something about that you must really value (*group member suddenly tears up.*)
Therapist:	(*pauses and holds the moment for a bit, then addresses another group member*) You dearly loved to dance…can you say what was important to you about that?
Group member 2:	(*also emotional*) Just being with the music, expressing music…I can't do that anymore.
Therapist:	So dancing was a way for you to express your love of music?
Group member 2:	That's right.
Therapist:	Again, this is where my mind gets very busy, telling me I've no right to say this to you. But out of respect for *my* values, I'm nonetheless going to ask you: *What now?* (*long pause as she lets this settle in*) You have every right to choose to stop engaging in life. It is hard to live with pain.
Group member 1:	But I don't want to stop. I still want a life.
Therapist:	(*leaning in, speaking to the group*) Wow. Can you hear how powerful that is? I. Want. A. Life. (*group is silent, taking this in*)
Therapist:	What if it's possible to have a life worth living *with* chronic pain? What if you can live a vital live, a life that reflects what you care most deeply about, *if* you are willing to pay that toll?

At this point the therapist has laid the groundwork for willingness, values, and committed action. It would be a reasonable time to pull out a tool such as the Mindful Action Plan to help members identify their values and develop goals in the service of those values.

Therapist:	I've just given you a worksheet designed to help you determine how you can start living your values *right now.* Notice that at the top of the handout is the sentence "I am here now, accepting the way I feel and noticing my thoughts, while doing what I care about." With that in mind, let's work together to fill this out in a way that reflects your commitment to living a meaningful life. [*The therapist anticipates that members will continue to struggle and uses this to further the work:*]
Group member 3:	You're asking me to accept the way I feel, and the way I feel is broken. I don't like feeling fragile. I'm not sure how I'm supposed to move forward in my life until I start feeling better about myself, and when I tell myself I am fragile, I just spin on thinking about that.
Therapist:	Okay. What if you accepted the ideas of *I'm broken; I'm fragile?* [*willingness*] Are fragile people allowed to be loving, caring, kind, and giving to others? These are qualities that you identified are important to you [*values*].
Group member 3:	Well, yeah, I guess. Actually, one of my closest friends is surviving paralysis from the waist down and she has all of those qualities.
Therapist:	It's interesting the difference in how you talk about your friend and yourself. You said she is "surviving paralysis" but that you are "fragile" and "broken." It's as though your mind is telling you "surviving paralysis" is acceptable, and "fragile" is not. [*Notice the therapist is getting at fusion, self-as-context, and acceptance here.*]
Therapist:	(*continuing after pausing to let that sink in*) But I'm excited about what you just said, that you recognize one can be physically compromised and still show up in the ways you admire [*willingness, values, committed action*].

All the core processes are in play in these example exchanges, but the consistent focus is on moving with one's feet in a valued direction.

Once everyone has completed the plan, or at least gotten a good start, the therapist solicits feedback regarding how members experienced the exercise. She wraps up the session by thanking members for how they showed up in the group and shares her hope that they will continue on the path toward vital living.

Though meaningful work can be done in only one ACT session, psychological flexibility is an ongoing process. These group members (like all of us) have a lifetime's worth of work ahead. Fortunately there are many ACT resources available including self-help books, online resources, and videos. We recommend providing participants with a list of such resources (see "Furthering Your ACT Skills," available at http://www.newharbinger.com/23994.)

Summary

This chapter tackled the formidable task of providing readers with a sense of the different ways ACT can be (and is) delivered in a group setting. The flexibility of the model defied categorization—for every "defining" clinical dimension there were exceptions; for every curriculum we put forth there were any number of others that would also suffice. ACT just doesn't fit in a box, no matter what size or shape. For this reason we focused on the clinical decision making involved in a sample of different types of groups. Of the innumerable possibilities, we selected or designed examples that provided a range of the clinical considerations a therapist might encounter. We hope this approach will help readers work through the considerations involved in tailoring ACT to the unique needs of their own groups.

There *is* a common denominator present in all these examples. Regardless of the setting, the population, or the many contextual variables that come into play, the core ACT processes are at the heart of the treatment. By consistently looking through that ACT lens, you too can harness the potential power of ACT in a way that works for your group.

Conclusion

As we wrap up this book about conducting ACT in groups, we find ourselves reflecting on basic human nature. We are such funny creatures! We are intensely social, yet we often feel alone. We have this languaging ability that gives us tremendous capabilities but that also weaves an intricate web of history, association, evaluation, and meaning so tightly around us we lose touch with others and even ourselves.

How fitting, then, that we break through that web in the context of a group. ACT is designed to help build the skills needed to loosen the grip of language so that we can move through the world in a way that is *open, centered*, and *engaged*. This is meaningful work indeed, and when it takes place in a group setting, the potential for genuine connection—in our suffering, in our humanity, and in our power to create lives with meaning—is simply huge.

Engaging in this work has offered us more than we can express. We hope those of you intending to conduct ACT in groups will find the same.

With gratitude,

—Darrah and Joann

Acknowledgments

From Joann:

To every person who has been in one of my groups—clients and trainees alike—I have learned the most about group work from you… Thank you. To Larry, who has never met an obstacle he can't shoulder and has always been my rock, and has massaged the rocks out of my shoulders… Thank you. To Darrah, my new sister, mentor, and mirror, all in equal measures, I am forever grateful for your wisdom, friendship, and compassion… Thank you.

From Darrah:

Thank you to the folks at New Harbinger for your tremendous patience and faith. To my coauthor and partner-in-crime: Joann, you epitomize grace and grit—two qualities I admire greatly. To Andrew, thank you for your support and never actually *saying* "I told you so." And to Chloe, who at 8, seemed to view this book as she would an attention-grabbing sibling, thanks for loving me anyway.

> *Chloe:*   What are you writing about now, Mama?
>
> *Me:*   I'm writing about how to have difficult feelings.
>
> *Chloe:*   (*authoritatively*) Just tell them sometimes we get sad but that's just natural.

Huh. That could have saved some time.

References

Dailey, R. M., Crook, B., Glowacki, E., Prenger, E., & Winslow, A. A. (2016). Meeting weight management goals: The role of partner confirmation. *Health Communication, 31*(12), 1482–1494. doi:10.1080/10410236.2015.1089398

Follette, V., & Pistorello, J. (2007). *Finding life beyond trauma: Using acceptance and commitment therapy to heal from post-traumatic stress and trauma-related problems.* Oakland, CA: New Harbinger Publications.

Hayes, S. C. (2005). *Get out of your mind and into your life: The new acceptance and commitment therapy.* Oakland, CA: New Harbinger Publications.

Hayes, S. C., Pankey, J., Gifford, E. V., Batten, S., & Quiñones, R. (2002). Acceptance and commitment therapy in the treatment of experiential avoidance disorders. In T. Patterson (Ed.), *Comprehensive handbook of psychotherapy: Cognitive-behavioral approaches* (Vol. 2, pp. 319–351). New York, NY: Wiley.

Hayes, S. C., Strosahl, K. D., & Wilson, K. J. (1999). *Acceptance and commitment therapy: An experiential approach to behavioral change.* New York, NY: Guilford Press.

Hayes, S. C., Strosahl, K. D., & Wilson, K. J. (2011). *Acceptance and commitment therapy: The process and practice of mindful change* (2nd ed.). New York, NY: Guilford Press.

Kabat-Zinn, J. (1994). *Wherever you go, there you are.* New York, NY: Hyperion.

McHugh, L., & Stewart, I. (2012). *The self and perspective taking: Contributions and applications from modern behavioral science.* Oakland, CA: New Harbinger Publications.

Moran, D. J. (2015). Using the Mindful Action Plan to Accelerate Performance in the Workplace. Invited address at the Association for Contextual Behavior Science Southeat Conference in Lafayette, LA.

Strosahl, K., Robinson, P., & Gustavsson, T. (2012). *Brief interventions for radical change: Principles and practice of focused acceptance and commitment therapy*. Oakland, CA: New Harbinger Publications.

Torneke, N. (2010). *Learning RFT: An introduction to relational frame theory and its clinical application*. Oakland, CA: New Harbinger Publications.

Villatte, M., Villatte, J., & Hayes, S. C. (2015). *Mastering the clinical conversation: Language as intervention*. New York, NY: The Guilford Press.

Walser, R. D., & Westrup, D. (2007). *Acceptance and commitment therapy for the treatment of post-traumatic stress disorder and trauma-related problems: A practitioner's guide to using mindfulness and acceptance strategies*. Oakland, CA: New Harbinger Publications.

Westrup, D. (2014). *Advanced acceptance and commitment therapy: The experienced practitioner's guide to optimizing delivery*. Oakland, CA: New Harbinger Publications.

Darrah Westrup, PhD, is a licensed clinical psychologist practicing in Colorado and California with an established reputation for her work as a therapist, program director, trainer, researcher, and consultant to practitioners at various firms and organizations. She is a recognized authority on post-traumatic stress disorder (PTSD) and acceptance and commitment therapy (ACT), and has conducted numerous presentations and trainings at international, national, and local conferences, seminars, and workshops. She served for over five years as an expert ACT consultant for the VA-wide evidence-based treatment rollout of ACT for depression, and is author of *Advanced Acceptance and Commitment Therapy*. Westrup has also coauthored two additional books on ACT: *Acceptance and Commitment Therapy for the Treatment of Post-Traumatic Stress Disorder and Trauma-Related Problems* and *The Mindful Couple*.

M. Joann Wright, PhD, is currently director of clinical training and anxiety services at Linden Oaks Behavioral Health at Edward Hospital in Naperville, IL. She is also executive director of the Psychological Solutions Institute in Lisle, IL. Prior to moving to the Chicago, IL, area, she was a faculty member at Hofstra University's psychology department. Wright is dedicated to teaching and delivering contextual behaviorally based, empirically-supported treatment strategies, protocols, and models in order to help people reduce the suffering in their lives. Wright has presented scholarly papers, workshops, and presentations at national and international psychological conferences.

Index

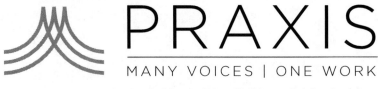

A subsidiary of New Harbinger Publications, Inc.

Enhance your practice with live ACT workshops

Praxis Continuing Education and Training—a subsidiary of New Harbinger Publications—is the premier provider of evidence-based continuing education for mental health professionals. Praxis specializes in ongoing **acceptance and commitment therapy (ACT)** training—taught by leading ACT experts. Praxis workshops are designed to help professionals learn and effectively implement ACT in session with clients.

ACT BootCamp®: Introduction to Implementation

For professionals with no prior experience with ACT, as well as those who want to refresh their knowledge

Learn the foundations of the psychological flexibility model, and develop a beginning set of skills in acceptance and commitment therapy (ACT). Understand the basics of relational frame theory (RFT)—the theory of language and cognition on which ACT is built. See, do, get feedback. Get hands-on, guided practice recognizing psychological inflexibility in clients in real time, and learn to fluidly respond from all points on the hexaflex. Dig into how ACT reinvigorates your therapeutic relationship with clients. Close with one day of practical review of what you've learned, reinforcing tools and techniques for working with clients. For total ACT immersion, attend evening sessions to learn from ACT experts to get your questions answered and build community.

ACT 1: Introduction to ACT

For professionals with no prior experience with ACT

Learn the foundations of the psychological flexibility model, and develop a beginning set of skills in acceptance and commitment therapy (ACT). See, do, get feedback. Dive into relational frame theory (RFT)—the theory of language and cognition on which ACT is built. Learn the hexaflex (flexible contact with the present moment, cognitive defusion, acceptance, self-as-context, values, committed action) and the basic processes of ACT while adding ACT metaphors and techniques to your therapeutic toolbox.

CONCEPTUAL | EXPERIENTIAL | PRACTICAL

ACT 2: Clinical Skills-Building Intensive

For professionals who practice ACT, but want more hands-on experience

This skills-building intensive includes round after round of interactive, experiential exercises. You will see, do, and get feedback as you build a solid basis in the dynamic use of acceptance and commitment therapy (ACT) interventions. The outcome? A better understanding of the model, and the ability to recognize inflexibility in clients and respond in real time. The net result: better clinical outcomes.

ACT 3: Mastering ACT

For professionals actively using ACT who want to apply it to their most complex cases

This master class is about the art and science of doing acceptance and commitment therapy (ACT) well with all of your clients. Bring your most difficult cases into the training, and work with master ACT trainers to resolve your biggest challenges. Develop an understanding of the intra- and interpersonal processes that happen inside the therapy room. Develop a deeper understanding of how your own behaviors impact yourself, as well as your clients in the therapy room. Get intensive practice conducting functional analysis in the moment, and then apply ACT solutions to your findings.

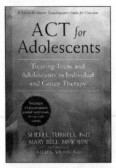
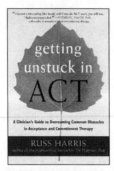
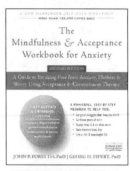
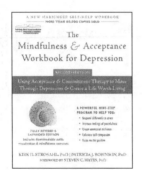
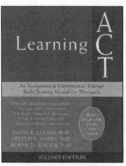
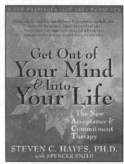

Register your **new harbinger** titles for additional benefits!

When you register your **new harbinger** title—purchased in any format, from any source—you get access to benefits like the following:

- Downloadable accessories like printable worksheets and extra content

- Instructional videos and audio files

- Information about updates, corrections, and new editions

Not every title has accessories, but we're adding new material all the time.

Access free accessories in 3 easy steps:

1. Sign in at NewHarbinger.com (or **register** to create an account).

2. Click on **register a book**. Search for your title and click the **register** button when it appears.

3. Click on the **book cover or title** to go to its details page. Click on **accessories** to view and access files.

That's all there is to it!

If you need help, visit:

NewHarbinger.com/accessories

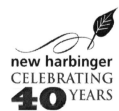

new harbinger
CELEBRATING
40 YEARS